Official Journal of the Federation of European Nutrition Societies (FENS)
Official Journal of the European Academy of Nutritional Sciences (EANS)

Annals of Nutrition & Metabolism

European Journal of Nutrition, Metabolic Diseases and Dietetics

Founded 1959 as 'Nutritio et Dieta' by E. Azerad, H. Kapp and J. Trémolières
Continued by A. Wretlind (1961–1969)
Continued by N. Zöllner (1970–1990) as 'Nutrition and Metabolism' (1970–1980), since 1980 integrating 'Annales de la Nutrition et de l'Alimentation', continued as 'Annals of Nutrition and Metabolism'
Continued by G. Wolfram (1991–1999)

KARGER

Printed in Switzerland
on acid-free paper by
Reinhardt Druck, Basel

Appears bimonthly:
1 volumes per year
(6 issues)

General Information

Annals of
Nutrition & Metabolism

Publication data: 'Annals of Nutrition and Metabolism' is published 6 times a year. Volume 49 with 6 issues appears in 2005.

Subscription rates: Subscriptions run for a full calendar year. Prices are given per year.

Personal subscription:

Print or Online	Print/Online combined
CHF 413.40	CHF 454.40
EUR 306.30	EUR 336.30
USD 375.90	USD 412.90
postage and handling	(added to print and print/online)
CHF 32.70 Europe,	CHF 48.60 Overseas
EUR 23.70	
USD 44.10	

Institutional subscription:

Print or Online	Print/Online combined
CHF 1378.–	CHF 1488.–
EUR 1021.–	EUR 1102.–
USD 1253.00	USD 1353.00
postage and handling	(added to print and print/online)
CHF 40.80 Europe,	CHF 60.60 Overseas
EUR 29.40	
USD 55.20	

Airmail surcharge: CHF 40.80 / USD 33.90

Discount subscription prices:
Federation of European Nutrition Societies (FENS) and European Academy of Nutritional Sciences (EANS)

Microforms: Please direct all enquiries and orders to:
University Microfilms Inc.
300 North Zeeb Road, P.O. Box 1346
Ann Arbor, MI 48106-1346 (USA)

Subscription orders: Orders can be placed at agencies, bookstores, directly with the Publisher
S. Karger AG, P.O. Box
CH–4009 Basel (Switzerland)
or with any of the following distributors:
Deutschland: S. Karger GmbH, Postfach
D–79095 Freiburg
France: Librairie Luginbühl
36, bd de Latour-Maubourg
F–75007 Paris
Great Britain, Ireland: S. Karger AG
4 Rickett Street
London SW6 1RU, UK
USA: S. Karger Publishers, Inc.
26 West Avon Road, P.O. Box 529
Farmington, CT 06085, USA
India, Bangladesh, Sri Lanka:
Panther Publishers Private Ltd.
33, First Main
Koramangala First Block
Bangalore 560 034, India
Japan: Karger Japan, Inc.
Yushima S Bld. 3F
4-2-3, Yushima, Bunkyo-ku
Tokyo 113-0034, Japan

Change of address: Both old and new address should be sent to the subscription source.

Single issues and back volumes: Information can be obtained through the Publisher.

Advertising: Correspondence and rate requests should be addressed to the Publisher.

Bibliographic indices: This journal is regularly listed in bibliographic services, including *Current Contents®* and Index Medicus/MEDLINE.

Copying: This journal has been registered with the Copyright Clearance Center (CCC), as indicated by the code appearing on the first page of each article. For readers in the US, this code signals consent for copying of articles for personal or internal use, or for the personal or internal use of specific clients, provided that the stated fee is paid per copy directly to
Copyright Clearance Center Inc.
222 Rosewood Drive
Danvers, MA 01923 (USA)
A copy of the first page of the article must accompany payment. Consent does not extend to copying for general distribution, for promotion, for creating new works, or for resale. In these cases, specific written permission must be obtained from the copyright owner,
S. Karger AG,
P.O. Box, CH–4009 Basel (Switzerland).

KARGER

Fax +41 61 306 12 34
E-Mail karger@karger.ch
www.karger.com

The Journal Home Page is available at:
www.karger.com/anm

F 05523

Annals of
Nutrition&
Metabolism

Promoting Fruit and Vegetable Consumption in Children across Europe – The Pro Children Project

Guest Editors
Johannes Brug, Rotterdam
Agneta Yngve, Stockholm
Knut-Inge Klepp, Oslo

12 figures and 26 tables, 2005

KARGER

Basel · Freiburg · Paris · London · New York ·
Bangalore · Bangkok · Singapore · Tokyo · Sydney

S. Karger
Medical and Scientific Publishers
Basel • Freiburg • Paris • London
New York • Bangalore • Bangkok
Singapore • Tokyo • Sydney

P.O. Box, CH–4009 Basel (Switzerland)
Printed in Switzerland on acid-free paper by
Reinhardt Druck, Basel
ISBN 3–8055–8018–5

KARGER

Fax +41 61 306 12 34
E-Mail karger@karger.ch
www.karger.com

Vol. 49, No. 4, 2005

Annals of Nutrition & Metabolism

Contents

KARGER

Fax +41 61 306 12 34
E-Mail karger@karger.ch
www.karger.com

Access to full text and tables of contents, including tentative ones for forthcoming issues: www.karger.com/anm_issues

Editorial

Annals of Nutrition & Metabolism

Ann Nutr Metab 2005;49:209–211
DOI: 10.1159/000087244

Published online: July 28, 2005

The Pro Children Study: Conceptualization, Baseline Results and Intervention Development of a European Effort to Promote Fruit and Vegetable Consumption in Schoolchildren

Johannes Brug[a] Agneta Yngve[b] Knut-Inge Klepp[c]

[a]Department of Public Health, Erasmus University Medical Center Rotterdam, Rotterdam, The Netherlands;
[b]Unit for Preventive Nutrition, Karolinska Institute, Stockholm, Sweden;
[c]Department of Nutrition, Faculty of Medicine, University of Oslo, Oslo, Norway

There is international consensus that a high fruit and vegetable intake is good for health; increasing fruit and vegetable consumption is one of the main dietary recommendations in the World Health Organization's global strategy on diet, physical activity and health [1] and fruit and vegetable promotion is likewise part of health promotion goals in many countries [2]. This is not surprising because fruits and vegetables are a primary source of diverse micronutrients and minerals, nonnutrient antioxidants and dietary fibers. Furthermore, a large body of evidence shows that an ample amount of fruit and vegetable in the daily diet contributes to lower risks for cardiovascular disease [3], cancer [4] (but see Hung et al. [5] for recent evidence that the cancer prevention effects of fruit and vegetable may be more doubtful), and obesity [6].

Nowadays, health promotion should be the result of careful planning [7, 8]. Following a thorough epidemiological analysis that identifies the health behaviors that importantly help to prevent major public health threats, the prevalence of such behavior and differences in these risk behaviors across populations should be studied in order to identify priority target groups. The next step is to identify the personal and environmental determinants of these behaviors in these priority groups, and to develop and pretest interventions that are tailored to these determinants. Finally, these interventions need to be implemented and disseminated in settings that ensure optimal exposure, and the intervention effects need to be evaluated. To go through these steps takes time and effort, and often interventions are implemented without such a proper development and testing process.

The Pro Children consortium was offered the opportunity, based on funding by the European Commission, to carefully develop a school-based fruit and vegetable promotion program aimed at 11- to 13-year-old children across Europe. The Pro Children Project was invented and is being conducted by a multidisciplinary team of researchers trained in human nutrition, health education and health promotion, epidemiology, community medicine, public health, sociology, psychology and biochemistry from 9 European countries. The Pro Children Project is thus an ambitious attempt to take all the necessary steps to develop, implement and evaluate evidence- and theory-driven promotion of fruit and vegetable consumption in primary schoolchildren in Europe. This special issue of *Annals of Nutrition and Metabolism* presents a series of papers on the important first steps within the Pro Children Project. In these initial stages of the Pro Children Project, a first study was conducted to develop and

KARGER

Fax +41 61 306 12 34
E-Mail karger@karger.ch
www.karger.com

0250–6807/05/0494–0209$22.00/0

Accessible online at:
www.karger.com/anm

Johannes Brug, PhD
Department of Public Health, Erasmus MC
University Medical Center Rotterdam, PO Box 2730
NL–3000 DR Rotterdam (The Netherlands)
Tel. +31 10 4087714, Fax +31 10 4089455, E-Mail j.brug@erasmusmc.nl

validate the much needed questionnaires applicable across countries to assess fruit and vegetable intake levels and determinants of intakes in children and their parents [9, 10]; next, focus groups [11] and personal interviews with children, parents and teachers were conducted to explore determinants of fruit and vegetable intake in children as well as possible intervention strategies to address these determinants; finally, cross-sectional survey studies were done to investigate intake levels [12, 13] and potential determinants of intakes [14] in children and their parents in 9 European countries. All these studies provided important input for the development of a school-based fruit and vegetable promotion program [15]. This program was pretested and is being implemented and evaluated.

In the first paper in this issue, Klepp et al. [16] present the rationale and the theoretical framework for the Pro Children study. The conclusion from that paper is that Europe with its large variation in intakes and food environments provides an especially interesting setting for investigating differences in intakes, determinants of intakes and intervention strategies related to fruits and vegetables. The authors further build a case for using schools as the main channel for fruit and vegetable promotion in children, since schools provide the opportunity to influence personal, as well as the social and physical environmental determinants of children's fruit and vegetable intake.

Dietary change interventions should build on up-to-date evidence of current intake levels, but no truly comparable data on fruit and vegetable intake in 11- to 13-year-old children or their parents across Europe were available before the Pro Children study, and easy-to-administer measurement instruments applicable in schools in different European countries to collect such data had to be developed. Haraldsdóttir et al. [10] report on the development and validity of self-administered teacher-guided 24-hour recall and food frequency questionnaires for 11- to 13-year-old children. They conclude that the validity of the food frequency questionnaire is acceptable with respect to ranking of the children based on their fruit and vegetable intake. This is of critical importance when investigating potential correlates of individual intake levels. With respect to the assessment of the absolute level of intake at the group level based on the 24-hour recall, there was a tendency to overestimation. Thus, the applied 24-hour format assessment method was adjusted prior to the implementation of the main study.

These instruments were subsequently used to explore fruit and vegetable intake across Europe. Yngve et al. [12] report on intakes in children, while Wolf et al. [13] report on their mothers' intakes. The results of both papers clearly show that fruit and vegetable intakes are indeed lower than public health recommendation in all Pro Children countries, especially when fruit juice is not included in the overall intake levels.

Since low intakes are so prevalent, there is a need for effective interventions, and it is therefore important to study potential determinants of intake. Wind et al. [11] present results from focus groups held in 2 of the Pro Children countries to explore why children eat or do not eat plenty of fruit and vegetable, and their study was also used to shape the Pro Children questionnaire. Sandvik et al. [14] present a quantitative description of children's motivations, abilities and opportunities to eat fruit and vegetable in all 9 participating countries. Both studies indicate that children in Europe have positive attitudes toward fruit and vegetable, most so for fruit. Both papers also stress the importance of increasing the availability and accessibility of fruit and vegetable, especially in the school environment.

Based on this evidence and additional literature studies, Pérez-Rodrigo et al. [15] give a detailed description of the rationale, goals and contents of the Pro Children intervention program.

The present set of Pro Children papers sets the stage, but the real 'proof of the pudding is in the eating'. Ongoing evaluation research will show if the Pro Children intervention can contribute to adoption of healthier diets in European schoolchildren, but also provide important information concerning the opportunities and constraints with respect to implementing school-based intervention strategies across Europe.

References

1 World Health Organization: Global strategy on diet, physical activity and health. 2005. http://www.who.int/dietphysicalactivity/en/.

2 World Health Organization: Promoting fruit and vegetable consumption around the world. 2005. http://www.who.int/dietphysicalactivity/fruit/en/.

3 Srinath Reddy K, Katan MB: Diet, nutrition and the prevention of hypertension and cardiovascular diseases. Public Health Nutr 2004;7: 167–186.

4 Key TJ, Schatzkin A, Willett WC, Allen NE, Spencer EA, Travis RC: Diet, nutrition and the prevention of cancer. Public Health Nutr 2004; 7:187–200.

5 Hung HC, Joshipura KJ, Jiang R, Hu FB, Hunter D, Smith-Warner SA, Colditz GA, Rosner B, Spiegelman D, Willett WC: Fruit and vegetable intake and risk of major chronic disease. J Natl Cancer Inst 2004;96:1577–1584.

6 Swinburn BA, Caterson I, Seidell JC, James WP: Diet, nutrition and the prevention of excess weight gain and obesity. Public Health Nutr 2004;7:123–146.

7 McKenzie JF, Smeltzer JL: Planning, Implementing, and Evaluating Health Promotion Programs: A Primer, ed 3. Boston, Allyn and Bacon, 2001.

8 Brug J, Oenema A, Ferreira I: Theory, evidence and intervention mapping to improve behavioral nutrition and physical activity interventions. Int J Behav Nutr Phys Act 2005; 2:2.

9 De Bourdeaudhuij I, Klepp K-I, Wind M, Due P, Brug J: Reliability of a questionnaire to measure personal, social and environmental correlates of fruit and vegetable intake in 10- to 11-year-old children in 5 European countries. Public Health Nutr 2005;8:189–200.

10 Haraldsdóttir J, Thórsdóttir I, de Almeida MDV, Maes L, de Rodrigues C, Elmadfa I, Andersen LF: Validity and reproducibility of a precoded questionnaire to assess fruit and vegetable intake in European 11- to 12-year-old schoolchildren. Ann Nutr Metab 2005;49: 221–227.

11 Wind M, Bobelijn K, De Bourdeaudhuij I, Klepp K-I, Brug J: A qualitative exploration of determinants of fruit and vegetable intake among 10- and 11-year-old schoolchildren in the Low Countries. Ann Nutr Metab 2005;49:228–235.

12 Yngve A, Wolf A, Poortvliet E, Elmadfa I, Brug J, Ehrenblad B, Franchini B, Haraldsdóttir J, Krølner R, Maes L, Pérez-Rodrigo C, Sjöström M, Thórsdóttir I, Klepp K-I: Fruit and vegetable intake in a sample of 11-year-old children in 9 European countries: the Pro Children cross-sectional survey. Ann Nutr Metab 2005;49:236–245.

13 Wolf A, Yngve A, Elmadfa I, Poortvliet E, Ehrenblad B, Pérez-Rodrigo C, Thórsdóttir I, Haraldsdóttir J, Brug J, Maes L, de Almeida MDV, Krølner R, Klepp K-I: Fruit and vegetable intake of mothers of 11-year-old children in nine European countries: the Pro Children cross-sectional survey. Ann Nutr Metab 2005;49:246–254.

14 Sandvik C, De Bourdeaudhuij I, Due P, Brug J, Wind M, Bere E, Pérez-Rodrigo C, Wolf A, Elmadfa I, Thórsdóttir I, de Almeida MDV, Yngve A, Klepp K-I: Personal, social and environmental factors regarding fruit and vegetable intake among schoolchildren in 9 European countries – The Pro Children Study. Ann Nutr Metab 2005;49:255–266.

15 Pérez-Rodrigo C, Wind M, Hildonen C, Bjelland M, Aranceta J, Klepp K-I, Brug J: The Pro Children Intervention: applying the intervention mapping protocol to develop a school-based fruit and vegetable promotion programme. Ann Nutr Metab 2005;49:267–277.

16 Klepp K-I, Pérez-Rodrigo C, De Bourdeaudhuij I, Due P, Elmadfa I, Haraldsdóttir J, König J, Sjöström M, Thórsdóttir I, de Almeida MDV, Yngve A, Brug J: Promoting fruit and vegetable consumption among European schoolchildren: rationale, conceptualization and design of the Pro Children Project. Ann Nutr Metab 2005;49:212–220.

Annals of
Nutrition & Metabolism

Ann Nutr Metab 2005;49:212–220
DOI: 10.1159/000087245

Published online: July 28, 2005

Promoting Fruit and Vegetable Consumption among European Schoolchildren: Rationale, Conceptualization and Design of the Pro Children Project

Knut-Inge Klepp[a] Carmen Pérez-Rodrigo[b] Ilse De Bourdeaudhuij[c] Pernille Due[d] Ibrahim Elmadfa[e] Jóhanna Haraldsdóttir[f] Jürgen König[g] Michael Sjöström[h] Inga Thórsdóttir[i] Maria Daniel Vaz de Almeida[j] Agneta Yngve[h] Johannes Brug[k]

[a]Department of Nutrition, Faculty of Medicine, University of Oslo, Oslo, Norway; [b]Community Nutrition Unit, Department of Public Health, Bilbao, Spain; [c]Department of Movement and Sport Sciences, Ghent University, Ghent, Belgium; [d]Department of Social Medicine, University of Copenhagen, Copenhagen, Denmark; [e]Institute for Nutritional Sciences, University of Vienna, Vienna, Austria; [f]Research Department of Human Nutrition, Royal Veterinary and Agricultural University, Copenhagen, Denmark; [g]Institute of Food, Nutrition and Human Health, Massey University, Palmerston North, New Zealand; [h]Unit for Preventive Nutrition, Karolinska Institute, Stockholm, Sweden; [i]Unit for Nutrition Research, Landspitali University Hospital, Reykjavik, Iceland; [j]Faculty of Nutrition and Food Sciences, University of Porto, Porto, Portugal; [k]Department of Public Health, Erasmus University Medical Center Rotterdam, Rotterdam, The Netherlands

Key Words
Fruit consumption · Vegetable consumption · European schoolchildren and parents

Abstract
Background/Aims: The Pro Children Project was designed to assess fruit and vegetable consumption in European schoolchildren and their parents, as well as determinants of the children's consumption patterns. A second objective was to develop and test strategies, applicable across Europe, for promoting consumption of fruits and vegetables among schoolchildren and their parents. In this paper, the rationale, theoretical background, overall design and implementation of the project is presented. ***Methods:*** Surveys of national, representative samples of 11-year-old schoolchildren and their parents were conducted in 9 countries, i.e. in Austria, Belgium, Denmark, Iceland, the Netherlands, Norway, Portugal, Spain and Sweden. Comprehensive school-based educational programmes have been developed and tested in three settings, i.e. in Spain, the Netherlands and in Norway. A precoded 24-hour recall form combined with a set of food frequency questions assessing regular intake were used to assess fruit and vegetable consumption. Determinants were assessed employing a comprehensive theoretical framework including personal, social and environmental factors related to fruit and vegetable consumption. The intervention programmes have been tested employing a group-randomized trial design where schools have been randomly allocated to an intervention arm and a delayed intervention arm. Surveys among all participating children and their parents were conducted prior to the initiation of the intervention, immediately after the end of the intervention and at the end of the subsequent school year. ***Conclusion:*** The project is expected to provide new information of great importance for improving our un-

KARGER

Fax +41 61 306 12 34
E-Mail karger@karger.ch
www.karger.com

0250–6807/05/0494–0212$22.00/0

Accessible online at:
www.karger.com/anm

Knut-Inge Klepp
Department of Nutrition
University of Oslo, Box 1046 Blindern
NO–0316 Oslo (Norway)
Tel. +47 22851378, Fax +47 22851531, E-Mail k.i.klepp@medisin.uio.no

derstanding of consumption patterns of fruits and vegetables and for guiding future efforts to promote increased consumption patterns across Europe.

Introduction

There is an international consensus that a high intake of fruit and vegetable promotes health by contributing to preventing severe public health problems such as cardiovascular diseases, obesity and a number of cancers [1–4]. However, the exact biological mechanisms largely remain unknown. Across Europe, there is great heterogeneity in the consumption patterns of vegetables and fruits both between regions and countries and within countries [5]. Large population groups, particularly in northern Europe, eat far less than the amount of vegetables and fruits recommended [5]. In southern Europe, it is of great concern that the previously seen variety, but also the overall intake of vegetables seems to be diminishing [6]. This heterogeneity is evident even at a young age as illustrated by the fact that while 58 and 52% of Portuguese 11-year-old girls and boys, respectively, reported eating fruit every day in 2001/2002, the corresponding figures among Flemish-speaking schoolchildren in Belgium were 33 and 27%, respectively [7]. For vegetables, the Flemish 11-year-olds, however, had the highest proportion of daily consumers (56 and 47% for girls and boys, respectively), while only 14% of Spanish children (both gender) reported eating vegetables every day according to the Health Behaviour in School-Aged Children study [7]. The fact that the large majority of schoolchildren (1–15 years old) report not eating fruit or vegetables every day indicates that this population segment consumes far less than what is recommended [7].

Children are at an age when habits, sometimes maintained throughout life, are learned and interventions aimed at children may thus have a lifelong impact [8, 9]. The large majority of children can effectively be reached through schools – an appropriate arena for health promotion. In addition, parents of schoolchildren constitute an important target group, as they importantly define most of their children's eating environment. Parents themselves constitute a large and important segment of the general population and previous nutrition education research indicates that parents can be reached through their children [10]. As a result, increasing the fruit and vegetable consumption and maintaining a large variety of these foods in the diet of Europeans are important health-related policy objectives of the European Union [1, 11].

In order to design effective interventions to increase the amount of vegetables and fruits eaten by children and adolescents, the mediators or determinants of consumption patterns need to be identified, as well as acceptable intervention strategies that can effectively change such mediators [12]. While there is an international body of research on this topic (primarily from the USA), such information has until recently largely been lacking for European child and adolescent population groups. Through literature searches, we have been able to identify a total of 20 published European studies investigating factors associated with fruit and/or vegetable intake among children and adolescents (see Rasmussen et al. [13] for an extensive review). Similarly, we have been able to identify 14 published European intervention studies designed to promote healthy eating habits among children and adolescents [14–27], of which only 3 were designed specifically to increase fruit and vegetable consumption [14, 15, 20]. To date, there have been no cross-European studies focusing on determinants of fruit and vegetable consumption in children and their parents. Furthermore, we are not aware of any multisite studies investigating the effectiveness of conceptually similar school-based nutrition intervention programmes across countries.

The purpose of this paper was to present the background, conceptualization and design of the Pro Children Project ('Promoting and Sustaining Health through Increased Vegetable and Fruit Consumption among European Schoolchildren') in progress in 9 European countries.

School-Based Nutrition Programmes

A major literature review of nutrition education programmes in school settings published in 1982 [28] concluded that 'we found it surprising that an area with such great preventive potential has produced so few empirical studies' and 'there is obviously a need for more and better research in nutrition education'. In 1992, a review of the research studies conducted during the 1980s concluded that there had been an increase in school-based nutrition education research over the past decade, and that 'research designs and methodologies have been greatly improved, compared with previous reviews' [29]. A comprehensive review of nutrition education research published in 1995 concluded that the following elements are critical with respect to effectiveness of nutrition education for schoolchildren [30]: (1) nutrition education is more likely to be effective when it is behaviourally focused; (2) nutrition education interventions are more likely to be effective when they employ educational strategies that are directly relevant to a behavioural focus and are derived from appropriate theory and research; (3) interventions need to devote adequate time and intensity to nutrition education to be effective; (4) family involvement enhances the effectiveness of programmes for younger children; (5) incorporation of self-evaluation or self-assessment and feedback is effective in interventions for older children; (6) effective nutrition education includes intervening in the school environment, and (7) interventions in the larger community can enhance school nutrition education.

These recommendations have been supported by more recent reviews [31–33]. In 1993, the National Cancer Institute in the United States began the '5 a Day for Better Health' initiative to increase fruit and vegetable consumption nationwide [34]. Nine community interventions were funded within this initiative, and 4 of them were school-based interventions for children/adolescents [35–38]. Three of these studies reported positive effects in the range of 0.2–0.6 servings of fruit and vegetable (or 9–12% increase compared to the comparison groups) [35–37]. The fourth study, the 'Alabama High 5 Project', reported a much larger effect (1.7 servings or 66% of adjusted total fruit and vegetable intake at baseline) [38]. An important difference between the High 5 Project and the other studies was that while the first 3 relied on regular classroom teachers to implement the programmes, the High 5 Project used trained staff ('curriculum coordinators'). While these '5 a Day' studies are clearly based on the current state-of-the-art recommendations, their effects appear, with one notable exception [38], to be modest. One possible explanation for the limited impact of these '5 a Day' campaigns could be their focus on cognitive and practical barriers to eating behaviour change [39]. Elsewhere, it has been pointed out that studies optimizing external validity by targeting diverse populations, including populations at risk, may lead to interventions being less flexible and responsive to the social and cultural environments within which they occur [40].

In Europe, the WHO's Health Promotion initiative [41] has inspired a number of school-based initiatives, including the European Network of Health Promoting Schools [42] and nutrition-specific efforts [43]. The strength of this comprehensive health promotion approach is its focus on empowerment, both at an individual (student) level through the development of personal skills, as well as on a local (school and community) level through health-promoting policies and supportive environments, thus increasing the abilities, as well as opportunities for health behaviour change.

Finally, over the past few years, making fruit and vegetables better available to children has been acknowledged as an important determinant of consumption patterns [44–46]. A recent paper reviewing the available literature on the school food environment concluded that environmental change interventions in schools show potential for positively affecting fruit and vegetable consumption among youth [47]. Thus, it was recommended that environmental strategies to increase the availability of vegetables and fruits and to support their choice by pupils be identified.

Pro Children Project

Given the rationale above, the Pro Children Project was designed to provide information on actual consumption levels of vegetables and fruits in European schoolchildren and their parents, to understand the determinants of consumption patterns among the children, and to develop and test effective strategies to promote adequate consumption levels of fruits and vegetables among schoolchildren. The specific research objectives are presented in table 1.

The project consists of two phases. In the first phase, relevant information for the planned development and implementation of fruit- and vegetable-promoting interventions is gathered. In the second phase, the planned interventions are developed, implemented and evaluated in group-randomized field studies. The first phase is conducted in 9 participating countries, i.e. in Austria, Belgium, Denmark, Iceland, the Netherlands, Norway, Portugal, Spain and Sweden, while the second phase is restricted to 3 countries, i.e. Spain, the Netherlands and Norway, as efficacy will have to be established prior to broader dissemination.

Assessing Consumption and Determinants

Comprehensive survey instruments assessing fruit and vegetable consumption and psychosocial factors associated with these consumption patterns have been developed for both pupils and their parents. Furthermore, a school staff survey instrument has been developed to assess school level opportunities and barriers related to fruit and vegetable consumption.

Table 1. Specific objectives of the Pro Children Project

Assessing fruit and vegetable consumption and correlates of consumption levels
To develop valid and reliable instruments for assessing fruit and vegetable consumption among schoolchildren and parents
To develop valid and reliable instruments for identifying factors influencing consumption patterns among schoolchildren
To determine the consumption levels of fruits and vegetables among schoolchildren and their parents in participating countries and in various subgroups (such as gender, socio-economic groups and cultural background)
To determine factors influencing the consumption of fruits and vegetables among schoolchildren in participating countries and in various subgroups (such as gender, socio-economic groups and cultural background)
To determine cross-national differences in fruit and vegetable consumption among children and their parents, as well as determinants of fruit and vegetable consumption among children
To determine the local, regional and national policies and organisational structures (including school meals) related to fruit and vegetable consumption
Design, implementation and evaluation (process, impact and efficacy) of the intervention programme
To design culturally relevant, but theoretically similar intervention programmes to be implemented in 3 participating countries
To determine facilitating and inhibiting factors for implementing the planned interventions
To determine how the various intervention components are perceived by the target groups (i.e. children and parents), as well as by other relevant actors (including teachers, school health personnel, local fruit and vegetable producers and distributors)
To determine to what extent the various intervention components are being implemented as planned
To determine whether the intervention produce the expected increase in fruit and vegetable consumption
To determine whether the intervention is equally effective in producing change across countries and within countries (in different demographic groups such as gender and socio-economic groups)
To determine whether changes in the identified theoretical factors account for the observed changes in fruit and vegetable consumption
To determine the cost-effectiveness of such an intervention programme

Fruit and Vegetable Consumption

In order to identify psychosocial factors associated with the fruit and vegetable intake at an individual level as well as to determine the effect of the intervention at a group level, it was decided to include both food frequency items and a 24-hour recall assessment in the survey instrument. Multiple pilot tests, including reliability and validity testing, were conducted in a number of countries before the final instrument was decided upon. Based on formal testing of the child instrument in Belgium, Denmark, Iceland, Norway, Portugal and Spain, it was concluded that the instrument was satisfactory with respect to ranking children according to their usual intake. However, the average intake, based on the 24-hour recall part, tended to overestimate the actual intake [48]. Formal testing of the parallel parental instrument indicated that the precoded 24-hour recall may be a valuable tool for measuring average intake of fruits and vegetables among adults. Moreover, the food frequency questionnaire was valid for ranking individuals according to their customary intake [49].

Psychosocial Determinants

Reviewing the research literature on predictors of fruit and vegetable intake among children and adolescents, it was concluded that there is a need to apply theory in a more systematic manner as well as to apply standardized instruments across diverse food-related cultural settings [13]. Furthermore, in line with state-of-the-art health promotion that takes a problem-driven approach, we included constructs from different behavioural theories in the Pro Children studies, to ensure inclusion of potential determinants at the individual, social and environmental level. Social cognitive theory [50], the 'attitude, social influences, self-efficacy model' [51], the theory of triadic influence [52], as well as a social-ecological perspective on health behaviour [53] were explored to develop the theoretical framework for the Pro Children project. This framework (fig. 1) guided both the development of the research instruments and the intervention.

This conceptual framework proposes that determinants of fruit and vegetable consumption can be found in the cultural, the physical and the social environment, and that they in turn influence the more proximal factors to be found at the personal level. Especially for children, who may have limited food choice autonomy, environmental factors such as fruit and vegetable availability may also more directly influence their intake. Thus, the model proposes that by introducing or clarifying more positive consequences of fruit and vegetable intake, by creating or encouraging a positive social environment and by making fruits and vegetables as easily available as possible at various arenas where the children spend their time, higher intentions and subsequent consumption of fruits and vegetables can be reached.

A similar process as for the intake instrument was performed in order to pilot and test the instrument assessing factors seen as important determinants of intake according to our conceptual framework. It was concluded that

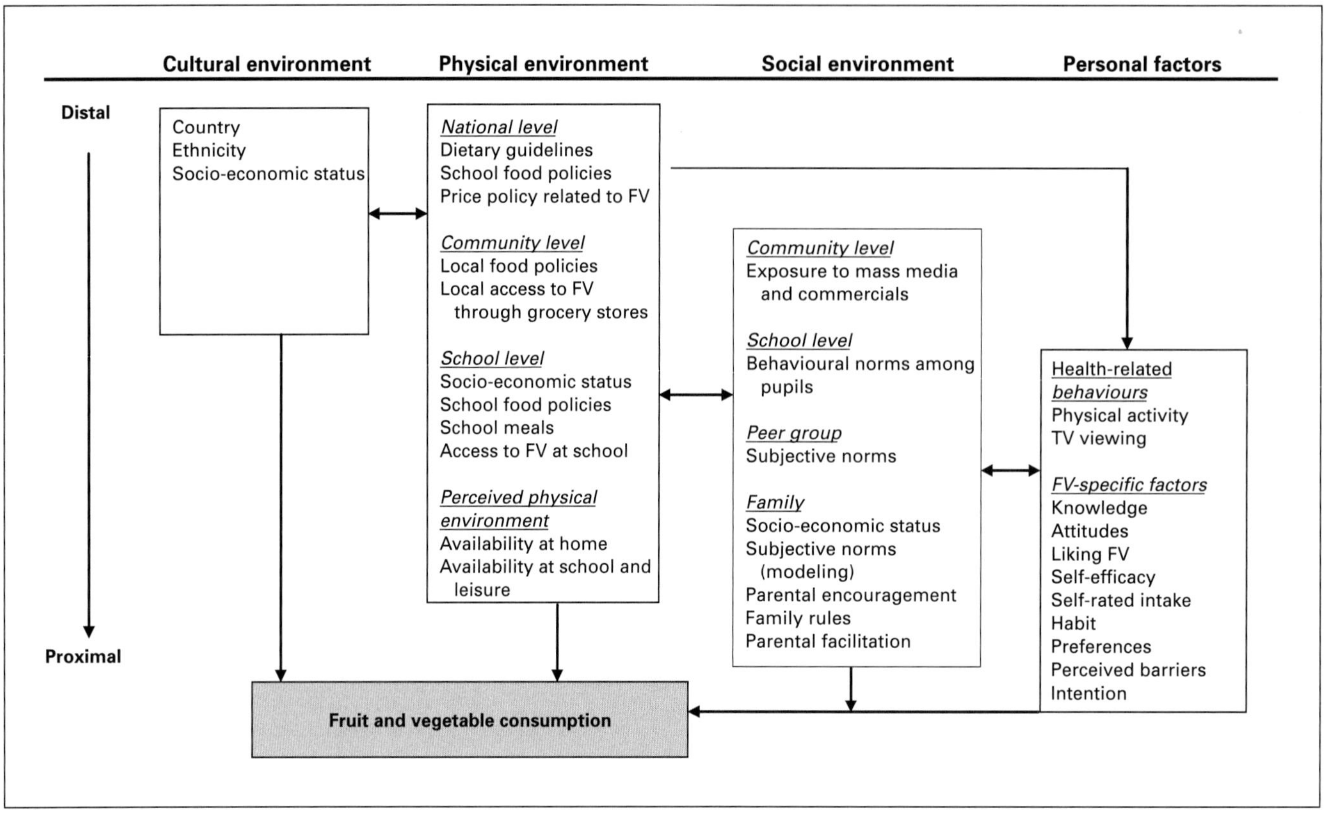

Fig. 1. Theoretical framework applied to children's fruit and vegetable (FV) consumption: the Pro Children Project.

the questionnaire provides a reliable and valid tool for assessing personal, social and environmental correlates of fruit and vegetable intake in 10- to 11-year-olds [54].

National, Cross-Sectional Surveys

The final survey instruments included the full assessment instrument and the determinant part for pupils and their parents, respectively. The instruments were originally developed in English prior to translation into the relevant languages within each participating country. These national versions were then back-translated into English by experts fluent in both English and the local language, but who were not involved in the development of the instruments. The back-translated versions were then compared to the original English version. Any inconsistencies were addressed and care was taken to secure comparability across languages in the final versions.

Surveys of 11-year-old schoolchildren and their parents were conducted in all 9 countries during October and November 2003 (table 2). National representative samples of schools were employed in each country with the exception of Austria (for Austria, the sample is representative for the Eastern region which includes 42% of the Austrian population) and Belgium (for Belgium, the sample is representative for Flanders, the Dutch-speaking part of Belgium). Schools constituted the sampling unit, and from each country samples of at least 20 schools and 1,300 eligible children were included. This student sample size was seen as sufficient to allow for the planned within-country comparisons (gender, socio-economic status and urban-rural differences) and taking the cluster sample into account.

The survey was, in all countries, administered by teachers. The questionnaires were completed during a 1- to 2-hour school session. Participating pupils received a questionnaire to take home and be completed by one of their parents. Pupil and parent questionnaires had pre-assigned identical code numbers to allow for subsequent linking of child-parent couples. The completed parent questionnaires were returned to the teachers who compiled and returned the questionnaires by mail to the research centres. The survey was conducted anonymously

Table 2. Pro Children Project; national cross-sectional surveys from October to November 2003: Participating countries, language groups, number of schools and participation rates

Country	Language	Schools	Eligible pupils	Participating pupils/ participation rate	Participating parents/ participation rate	School staff surveys/ participation rate
Austria	German	23	1,857	1,769 (95.3% of eligible)	1,574 (84.8% of eligible)	20 (87.0%)
Belgium	Flemish	50	1,604	1,355 (84.5%)	1,287 (80.2%)	50 (92.6%)
Denmark	Danish	59	2,111	1,942 (92.0%)	1,478 (70.0%)	59 (100.0%)
Iceland	Icelandic	32	1,392	1,235 (88.7%)	998 (71.7%)	32 (100.0%)
Netherlands	Dutch Turkish	49	1,396	1,113 (79.7%)	946 (67.8%)	49 (100.0 %)
Norway	Norwegian	52	1,347	1,205 (89.5%)	1,009 (74.9%)	51 (98.1%)
Portugal	Portuguese	27	2,535	2,494 (98.4%)	2,114 (83.4%)	19 (70.4%)
Spain	Basque, Catalan, Galician, Spanish	37	1,410	1,335 (94.7%)	1,089 (77.2%)	36 (97.3%)
Total	13	375	15,404	13,924 (90.4%)	11,727 (76.1%)	360 (95.0%)

in all countries, and prior research ethics clearance was obtained from all appropriate institutions.

Finally, a school staff survey instrument was developed and administered to the school headmasters (or the school staff person appointed by the headmaster) in order to assess school level opportunities and barriers related to fruit and vegetable consumption. In table 2, a listing of all countries with their respective languages, number of schools and participants, as well as participation rates for pupils, parents and school administrators is presented.

Pro Children Intervention Strategies

The intervention programmes build on the current state of the art within the healthy nutrition promotion tradition. Specifically, the programmes (1) focus on specific eating behaviours related to fruit and vegetable consumption; (2) employ educational strategies that are directly relevant to fruit and vegetable consumption and are derived from an appropriate theory for behavioural determinants; (3) devote adequate time and intensity in order to be effective; (4) include parental involvement and age-appropriate self-assessment and feedback in the form of computer-tailored feedback, and (5) include interventions targeting the school environment as well as the larger community.

In order to further advance the state of the art within the field of school-based public health nutrition intervention strategies, this approach is combined with the health promotion paradigm and attempts to utilise the cultural diversity and richness of Europe in designing the intervention strategies. Specifically, we (1) encourage local participation in planning and implementing the intervention to secure culturally relevant interventions and foster local ownership; (2) include sharing of relevant food habits across intervention sites in order to promote the European heterogeneity in terms of eating habits as a positive, motivational element for participants to explore; (3) conduct a cross-national test of the effectiveness of a comprehensive (theoretically similar, but culturally adapted) intervention approach.

The intervention programmes are designed to ensure approximately 20 h of exposure to food-based messages delivered to the children. These will be behaviour specific and the activities will provide opportunities for skill development during an 8-month period of intensive intervention followed by some booster activities the second year of intervention. The intervention in each of the 3 countries consists of core programme components, as well as additional, optional components that differ between the countries. In order to design the programmes, an adapted Intervention Mapping [55] process has been applied at all 3 sites. This process and the content of the intervention programmes is presented in detail elsewhere [56].

Evaluation Design

The intervention programmes are being tested in a group-randomized trial design where schools have been randomly allocated to an intervention arm and a delayed

Table 3. Evaluation design for the Pro Children intervention studies

Country/region	Schools	Baseline September 2003	Intervention October 2003 to April 2004	First follow-up May 2004	Cont. intervention September 2004 to April 2005	Second follow-up May 2005
Netherlands – Rotterdam area						
Intervention schools	12	10-year-olds and parents	core intervention	11-year-olds and parents	booster activities	12-year-olds and parents
Comparison schools	12	10-year-olds and parents		11-year-olds and parents		12-year-olds and parents
Norway – Buskerud County						
Intervention schools	9	11-year-olds and parents	core intervention	12-year-olds and parents	booster activities	13-year-olds and parents
Comparison schools	9	11-year-olds and parents		12-year-olds and parents		13-year-olds and parents
Spain – Bilbao region						
Intervention schools	10	10-year-olds and parents	core intervention	11-year-olds and parents	booster activities	12-year-olds and parents
Comparison schools	10	10-year-olds and parents		11-year-olds and parents		12-year-olds and parents

intervention arm (comparison group). Surveys among all participating children and their parents were conducted prior to the initiation of the intervention (September 2003; month 0), immediately after the end of the intervention (at month 8) and at the end of the subsequent school year (month 20). The design is presented in table 3. A cohort of children will thus be followed over a 20-month period from age 10–11 to age 12–13. The main comparisons will be between the intervention group and the comparison group at follow-up I and II, adjusted for baseline differences. The intervention study is taking place in 3 participating countries only, i.e. in the Bilbao region, Spain, in Rotterdam, the Netherlands, and in the Buskerud County of Norway. These settings represent different European regions, allowing us to test the intervention strategies in different cultural settings.

While the intensive intervention lasts only for one school year targeting 5th graders in the Netherlands and Spain (10- to 11-year-olds) and 6th graders in Norway (11- to 12-year-olds), we intend for the school- and community-based activities to be sustained. The degree to which this is actually the case is currently being investigated.

Primary nutrition-related outcomes are the amount (the specific objective is to obtain a 20% increase) and variety of vegetables and fruits consumed. Secondary targets are improvements in knowledge scores, attitudes, perceived social influence, self-efficacy, skills, perceived barriers, awareness indicators and availability of fruit and vegetable at school and at home.

In addition to the formative evaluation implicit in the Intervention Mapping approach [56] and the outcome evaluation, an extensive process evaluation is being conducted as part of the Pro Children intervention study. The process evaluation will include monitoring of the intervention delivery and perceived satisfaction and evaluation of the programmes by key actors. A thorough understanding of how the intervention is being implemented and perceived by the involved actors is critical in order to (1) guide the interpretation of observed outcome data, including secondary data analysis relating outcome to intervention exposure (amount and quality) and (2) identify important facilitating factors as well as barriers for successful intervention implementation.

Such information is seen as critical with respect to successful revisions and potential large-scale dissemination of the final Pro Children intervention programme. In addition, direct cost associated with the development, training and implementation of the intervention programmes will be monitored in order to allow for subsequent cost-effectiveness analyses. An overview of the various evaluation components included in the Pro Children Project is presented in table 4.

Table 4. Evaluation components included in the Pro Children Project

Formative evaluation
Literature review
Focus group discussions with children and parents
Pilot testing of intervention components
Feedback from teacher panels
Process evaluation
Classroom observation of programme implementation
Observation of available food, in particular vegetable and fruits at school
Community observation: proximity to food outlets; availability of vegetables and fruits
Media coverage of programme activities and fruit- and vegetable-related information
Teacher's feedback on programme activities (written and oral)
School administrators' feedback on programme activities
Pupils' assessment of programme activities (written as part of follow-up survey I and II and through focus group discussions
Cost assessment of programme development, training and implementation
Outcome evaluation
Baseline survey and follow-up surveys (at month 8 and month 20): assessment of amount and variety of vegetables and fruits consumed and determinants among pupils and parents
Baseline survey and follow-up surveys (at month 8 and month 20): assessment of fruit and vegetable availability at school, school food policies and guidelines as reported by school administrators

Conclusion

The large variation seen in eating habits across Europe, including practices related to the consumption of vegetables and fruit, makes it particularly interesting to conduct a study such as the Pro Children Project. We believe that the findings will be of great importance for improving our understanding of young consumers' acceptance, preferences, barriers and consumption patterns of vegetables and fruits. Such information is needed in order to better inform and guide effective intervention strategies.

Further information regarding the Pro Children study, including the computer-tailored programmes and published reports as they become available, can be found at the Pro Children Project's Web site: http://www.univie.ac.at/prochildren/.

Acknowledgement

This study is being carried out with financial support from the Commission of the European Communities, specific RTD programme 'Quality of Life and Management of Living Resources', QLK1-2001-00547 'Promoting and Sustaining Health through Increased Vegetable and Fruit Consumption among European Schoolchildren' (Pro Children). The study does not necessarily reflect the Commission's views and in no way anticipates the Commission's future policy in this area.

References

1 World Health Organization: Diet, Nutrition and the Prevention of Chronic Diseases. Report of a Joint WHO/FAO Expert Consultation. WHO Technical Report Series. Geneva, World Health Organization, 2003, No 916.
2 Hung H C, Joshipura KJ, Jiang R, Hu FB, Hunter D, et al: Fruit and vegetable intake and risk of major chronic disease. J Natl Cancer Inst 2004;96:1577–1584.
3 Paolini M, Sapone A, Canistro D, Antonelli MA, Chieco P: Diet and risk of cancer. Lancet 2003;361:257–258.
4 Maynard M, Gunnell D, Emmett P, Frankel S, Davey Smith G: Fruit, vegetables, and antioxidants in childhood and risk of adult cancer: The Boyd Orr cohort. J Epidemiol Community Health 2003;57:218–225.
5 Dafne (Data Food Networking) II: Network for the pan-European food data bank based on household budget surveys. Report from the European Commission and Agro-Industrial Research, Brussels, 1998.
6 Aranceta J, Pérez-Rodrigo C, Ribas L, Serra-Majem LI: Sociodemographic and lifestyle determinants of food patterns in Spanish children and adolescents: The enKid study. Eur J Clin Nutr 2003;57(suppl 1):S40–S44.
7 World Health Organization: Young People's Health in Context. Health Behaviour in School-Aged Children (HBSC) Study: International Report from the 2001/2002 Survey. Health Policy for Children and Adolescents, No 4. The Regional Office for Europe. Copenhagen, World Health Organization, 2004.
8 Kelder SH, Perry CL, Klepp K-I, Lytle L: Longitudinal tracking of adolescent smoking, physical activity and food choice behaviors. Am J Public Health 1994;84:1121–1126.
9 Lien N, Lytle LA, Klepp K-I: Stability in consumption of fruit, vegetables, and sugary foods in a cohort from age 14 to 21. Prev Med 2001; 33:217–226.
10 Perry CL, Luepker RV, Murray DM, Hearn MD, Halper A, Dudovitz B, Maile MC, Smyth M: Parent involvement with children's health promotion: A one-year follow-up of the Minnesota home team. Health Educ Q 1989;16: 1156–1160.
11 European Council: Council resolution of 14 December 2000 (2001/C 20/01) on health and nutrition. Official Journal of the European Communities, January 23, 2001.
12 Baranowski T, Cullen KW, Baranowski J: Psychosocial correlates of dietary intake: advancing dietary intervention. Ann Rev Nutr 1999; 19:17–40.
13 Rasmussen M, Krølner R, Klepp K-I, Lytle L, Brug J, Bere E, Due P: Determinants of fruit and vegetable consumption among children and adolescents: review of the literature. Submitted.
14 Bere E, Veierød MB, Klepp K-I: The Norwegian School Fruit Programme: Evaluating paid vs no-cost subscription. Prev Med 2005;41: 463–470.
15 Eriksen K, Haraldsdottir J, Pederson R, Flyger HV: Effect of a fruit and vegetable subscription in Danish schools. Public Health Nutr 2002;6: 57–63.
16 Friel S, Kelleher C, Campbell P, Nolan G: Evaluation of the Nutrition Education at Primary School (NEAPS) programme. Public Health Nutr 1999;2:549–555.

17 Hølund U: Promoting change of adolescent's sugar consumption: The 'Learning by Teaching' study. Health Educ Res 1990;5:451–458.
18 Klepp K-I, Wilhelmsen BU: Nutrition education in junior high schools: incorporating behavior change strategies into home economic courses. Health Educ Res 1993;8:547–554.
19 Klepp K-I, Øygard L, Tell GS, Vellar OD: Twelve-year follow-up study of a school-based health education program: The Oslo Youth Study. Eur J Public Health 1994;4:195–200.
20 Lowe CF, Horne PJ, Tapper K, Bowdery M, Egerton C: Effects of a peer modeling and rewards-based intervention to increase fruit and vegetable consumption in children. Eur J Clin Nutr 2004;58:510–522.
21 Manios Y, Kafatos A: Health and nutrition education in elementary schools: changes in health knowledge, nutrient intakes and physical activity over a six year period. Public Health Nutr 1999;2:445–448.
22 Manios Y, Moschandreas J, Hatzis C, Kafatos A: Evaluation of a health and nutrition education program in primary schoolchildren of Crete over a three-year period. Prev Med 1999; 28:149–159.
23 Moon AM, Mullee MA, Rogers L, Thompson RL, Speller V, Roderick P: Helping schools to become health-promoting environments – An evaluation of the Wessex Healthy School Award. Health Promot Int 1999;14:111–122.
24 Parker L, Fox A: The Peterborough Schools Nutrition Project: a multiple intervention programme to improve school-based eating in secondary schools. Public Health Nutr 2001;4: 1221–1228.
25 Perez-Rodrigo C, Aranceta J: Nutrition education for schoolchildren living in a low-income urban area in Spain. J Nutr Educ 1997;29:267–273.
26 Puska P, Vartiainen E, Pallonen U, Salonen JT, Poyhia P, Koskela K, McAlister A: The North-Karelia youth project: evaluation of two years of intervention on health behavior and CVD risk factors among 13- to 15-year-old children. Prev Med 1982;11:550–570.
27 Sahota P, Rudolf MCJ, Dizey R, Hill AJ Barth JH, Cade J: Evaluation of implementation and effect of primary school based intervention to reduce risk factors for obesity. BMJ 2001;323: 1027–1029.
28 Saylor KE, Coates TJ, Killen J, Slinkard LA: Nutrition education research: fast or famine?; in Coates TJ, Peterson AC, Perry C (eds): Promoting Adolescent Health. A Dialog on Research and Practice. New York, Academic Press, 1982, pp 355–380.
29 Contento IR, Manning AD, Shannon B: Research perspective on school-based nutrition education. J Nutr Educ 1992;24:247–260.
30 Contento I, Balch GI, Bronner YL, Lytle LA, Maloney SK, White SL, Olson CM, Swadener SS: The effectiveness of nutrition education and implications for nutrition education policy, programs, and research: a review of research. J Nutr Educ 1995;27:297–418.
31 Hoelscher DA, Evans A, Parcel GS, Kelder SH: Designing effective nutrition interventions for adolescents. J Am Diet Assoc 2002;102:S52–S63.
32 Ciliska D, Miles E, O'Brien MA, Turl C, Tomasik HH, Donovan U, Beyers J: Effectiveness of community-based interventions to increase fruit and vegetable consumption. J Nutr Educ 2000;32:341–352.
33 Pérez-Rodrigo C, Aranceta J: School-based nutrition education: lessons learned and new perspectives. Public Health Nutr 2001;41:131–139.
34 Havas S, Heimendinger J, Damron D, Nicklas TA, Cowan A, Beresford SAA, Sorensen G, Buller D, Bishop D, Baranowski T, Reynolds K: 5 a day for better health – 9 community research projects to increase fruit and vegetable consumption. Public Health Rep 1995;110: 68–79.
35 Baranowski T, Davis M, Resnicow K, Baranowski J, Doyle C, Lin LS, Smith M, Wang DT: Gimme 5 fruit, juice, and vegetables for fun and health: outcome evaluation. Health Educ Behav 2000;27:96–111.
36 Nicklas TA, Johnson CC, Myers L, Farris RP, Cunningham A: Outcomes of a high school program to increase fruit and vegetable consumption: gimme 5 – A fresh nutrition concept for students. J Sch Health 1998;68:248–253.
37 Perry CL, Bishop DB, Taylor G, Murray DM, Mays RW, Dudovitz BS, Smyth M, Story M: Changing fruit and vegetable consumption among children: the 5-a-Day Power Plus program in St Paul, Minnesota. Am J Public Health 1998;88:603–609.
38 Reynolds KD, Franklin FA, Binkley D, Raczynski JM, Harrington KF, Kirk KA, Person S: Increasing the fruit and vegetable consumption of fourth-graders: results from the high 5 project. Prev Med 2000;30:309–319.
39 Wardle J, Cooke LJ, Gibson EL, Sapochnik M, Sheiham A, Lawson M: Increasing children's acceptance of vegetables; a randomized trial of parent-led exposure. Appetite 2003;40:155–162.
40 Lytle LA, Jacobs DR Jr, Perry CL, Klepp K-I: Achieving physiological change in school-based intervention trials: what makes a preventive intervention successful? Invited commentary. Br J Nutr 202;88:219–221.
41 World Health Organization: Ottawa charter for health promotion. Health Promot 1986;1: iii–v.
42 World Health Organization: European Network of Health Promoting Schools. A Joint WHO-CE-CEC Project. Copenhagen, World Health Organization Regional Office for Europe, 1993.
43 World Health Organization: Healthy Nutrition: An Essential Element of a Health-Promoting School. WHO Global School Health Initiative. WHO Information Series on School Health. Geneva, World Health Organization, 1998.
44 Bere E, Klepp K-I: Correlates of fruit and vegetable intake among young adolescents: parental and self-reports. Public Health Nutr 2004; 7:991–998.
45 Cullen KW, Baranowski T, Owens E, Marsh T, Rittenberry L, de Moor C: Availability, accessibility, and preferences for fruit, 100% fruit juice, and vegetables influence children's dietary behavior. Health Educ Behav 2003;30: 615–626.
46 Neumark-Sztainer D, Wall M, Perry C, Story M: Correlates of fruit and vegetable intake among adolescents. Findings from Project EAT. Prev Med 2003;37:198–208.
47 French SA, Stables G: Environmental interventions to promote fruit and vegetable consumption among youth in school settings. Prev Med 2003;37:593–610.
48 Haraldsdóttir J, Thórsdóttir I, de Almeida MDV, Maes L, de Rodrigues C, Elmadfa I, Andersen LF: Validity and reproducibility of a precoded questionnaire to assess fruit and vegetable intake in European 11- to 12-year-old schoolchildren. Ann Nutr Metab 2005;49:221–227.
49 Kristjansdottir AG, Andersen LF, Haraldsdóttir J, de Almeida MDV, Thórsdóttir I: Validity of a questionnaire to assess fruit and vegetable intake in adults. Eur J Clin Nutr, submitted.
50 Bandura A: Self-Efficacy. The Exercise of Control. New York, Freeman, 1997.
51 Kok G, Schaalma H, De Vries H, Parcel G, Paulssen T: Social psychology and health education; in Stroebe W, Hewstone M (eds): European Review of Social Psychology. Chichester, Wiley, 1996, vol 7, pp 241–282.
52 Flay BR, Petraitis J: The theory of triadic influence: A new theory of health behavior with implications for preventive interventions; in Albrecht GS (ed): Advances in Medical Sociology. Reconsideration of Models of Health Behavior Change. Greenwich, JAI, 1994, vol 4, pp 19–44.
53 French SA, Story M, Jeffery RW: Environmental influences on eating and physical activity. Ann Rev Public Health 2001;22:309–335.
54 De Bourdeaudhuij I, Klepp K-I, Due P, Pérez-Rodrigo C, de Almeida MDV, Wind M, Krølner R, Sandvik C, Brug J: Reliability and validity of a questionnaire to measure personal, social and environmental correlates of fruit and vegetable intake in 10- to 11-year-old children in 5 European countries. Public Health Nutr 2005;8:189–200.
55 Bartholomew LK, Parcel GS, Kok G, Gottlieb NH: Intervention Mapping. Designing Theory- and Evidence-Based Health Promotion Programs. Mountain View, Mayfield Publishing Company, 2001.
56 Pérez-Rodrigo C, Wind M, Hildonen C, Bjelland M, Aranceta J, Klepp K-I, Brug J: The Pro Children intervention: applying the Intervention Mapping Protocol to develop a school-based fruit and vegetable promotion programme. Ann Nutr Metab 2005;49:267–277.

Annals of
Nutrition & Metabolism

Ann Nutr Metab 2005;49:221–227
DOI: 10.1159/000087276

Published online: July 28, 2005

Validity and Reproducibility of a Precoded Questionnaire to Assess Fruit and Vegetable Intake in European 11- to 12-Year-Old Schoolchildren

Jóhanna Haraldsdóttir[a] Inga Thórsdóttir[b,c] Maria Daniel Vaz de Almeida[d] Lea Maes[e] Carmen Pérez-Rodrigo[f] Ibrahim Elmadfa[g] Lene Frost Andersen[h]

[a]Department of Human Nutrition, Royal Veterinary and Agricultural University, Copenhagen, Denmark; [b]Unit for Nutrition Research, Landspitali University Hospital, and [c]Department of Food Science, University of Iceland, Reykjavik, Iceland; [d]Faculty of Nutrition and Food Sciences, University of Porto, Porto, Portugal; [e]Department of Public Health, Ghent University, Ghent, Belgium; [f]Community Nutrition Unit, Bilbao, Spain; [g]Institute for Nutritional Sciences, University of Vienna, Vienna, Austria; [h]Department of Nutrition, University of Oslo, Oslo, Norway

Key Words
Children · Fruit consumption · Validation · Vegetable consumption

Abstract
Background/Aims: Validity and reproducibility were evaluated of a new questionnaire to assess fruit and vegetable intakes in 11- to 12-year-old children. ***Methods:*** The precoded teacher-assisted self-administered questionnaire included two sections: a 24-hour recall part and a food frequency part. Validity was tested in 4 countries (Denmark, Iceland, Norway, Portugal; n = 43–60 per country) using a 1-day weighed food record and 7-day food records as reference methods. Test-retest (7–12 days apart) reproducibility was assessed in 6 countries (Belgium, Denmark, Iceland, Norway, Portugal, Spain; n = 60–74 per country). ***Results:*** Spearman rank correlations for fruit and vegetable intake according to the frequency part and the 7-day food record ranged between r = 0.40–0.53. Between 25–50% were classified into the same quartile and 70–88% into the same or adjacent quartile. Test-retest Spearman rank correlations for the food frequency part were r = 0.47–0.84. Three countries showed no significant difference between fruit intake as assessed with the 24-hour recall part and the 1-day weighed food record, and 2 countries showed no significant difference for vegetables. In the other countries, the 24-hour recall part resulted in substantially higher mean intake levels. ***Conclusion:*** Validity and reproducibility as to ranking of subjects were regarded to be satisfactory in all countries. Group mean intake, based on the original 24-hour part, was valid for fruit in 3 countries and for vegetables in 2 countries, and this part was subsequently adjusted to avoid overestimation, before the questionnaire was used in the Pro Children study.

Introduction

Consumption of fruit and vegetables in children in most European and North American countries is below the recommended intake of 400 g fruit and vegetable per day [1–3]. The Pro Children Project was set up to develop effective strategies to promote adequate consumption levels of fruit and vegetables among 11- to 13-year-old schoolchildren [4]. In the context of this project, valid and

KARGER
Fax +41 61 306 12 34
E-Mail karger@karger.ch
www.karger.com

0250–6807/05/0494–0221$22.00/0

Accessible online at:
www.karger.com/anm

Lene Frost Andersen
Department of Nutrition, University of Oslo
Box 1046, Blindern
NO–0316 Oslo (Norway)
Tel. +47 22851374, Fax +47 22851531, E-Mail l.f.andersen@medisin.uio.no

reliable instruments for assessing fruit and vegetable intake among schoolchildren had to be developed in order to be able to adequately describe consumption levels of fruit and vegetables across the 9 participating European countries and to measure the effect of the interventions.

A variety of methods for assessing habitual dietary intake are available, but most of these methods are time-consuming and cannot be used in large population samples. They also require a certain literacy level and motivation which make them difficult to use in young children. Difficulties in collecting accurate dietary intake data on children in large surveys have already been identified [5, 6]. Although the literature shows varying results of self-reported dietary assessment of schoolchildren, the food frequency questionnaire is increasingly being recognised as a suitable method for collecting data in epidemiological studies [5] from the age of 10 years and upwards when the cognitive processes of children become more similar to those of adults [6, 7]. Less is known about the use in children of a dietary recall method, like the 24-hour recall, when it is administered in the form of a questionnaire instead of as a personal interview.

For the Pro Children Project, a specific instrument for measuring fruit and vegetable intake had to be developed, suitable for collecting the information from 11- to 13-year-old children themselves, without the assistance of their parents, in a large survey including several thousands of children. It should also be suitable for use across Europe, i.e. in southern as well as northern European countries. The collected data should give valid information on the ranking of children related to their usual intake and on the mean intake of the group. The fruit and vegetable intake data are to be used (1) for investigating relationships between intake and potential determinants of intake, (2) for measuring the effect of an intervention study aiming at increasing intake and (3) for comparison of intake between the 9 European countries participating in the Pro Children Project. To date, only few studies have been published on the reliability and validity of dietary methods evaluating self-reports of fruit and vegetable intake among young children without the help of parents or interviewers [8–14].

The dietary questionnaire developed for this purpose includes two sections: a precoded 24-hour recall part and a food frequency part. The 24-hour part is used for measuring group mean intake and for specifying the type of fruit and vegetables eaten, whereas the food frequency part is used for ranking subjects according to their usual intake. The objective of the present study was to measure the validity and the reproducibility of this questionnaire.

Methods and Subjects

Validation Study: Design and Subjects

Validity was tested according to the same protocol in 4 countries (Denmark, Norway, Iceland and Portugal), using a 7-day food record as the reference method. The questionnaire was filled in by the children at school and the food record was started 1–8 days later. On the first recording day, all foods eaten were weighed on a scale (weighed food record), whereas during the following 6 days, the consumed quantities were described by household measures and standard units (estimated food record). This was done in order to reduce the burden on the participants and thus increase participation rate. The validity study was carried out in February to March 2003.

Subjects, 11-year-old boys and girls, were recruited through local schools and class teachers. None of the children had participated in any pretesting of the questionnaire. Participation was voluntary and the children had to present a written consent signed by one of their parents. Participation rates ranged between 31 and 43%. In Norway, 196 received an invitation letter, 65 completed the study but 5 had incomplete records. Data are presented for 60 participants (participation rate 31%). In Denmark, 151 children received an invitation letter, 59 children completed the study; 3 were excluded because of inconsistent data. Data are presented for 56 participants (participation rate 37%). In Iceland, 101 received an invitation letter, 62 completed the study, 19 were excluded because of incomplete records or because they were regarded as outliers (total intake of fruit and vegetables excluding juice >1,000 g/day). The data of 43 children were analysed (participation rate 43%). In Portugal, 137 received an invitation letter, 50 completed the study but 4 were excluded as outliers. Data are presented for 46 participants (participation rate 34%). Mean age was between 11.2 and 11.6 years (range 11–12 years). The percentage of girls were: Denmark 55%, Norway 47%, Iceland 65% and Portugal 54%.

Reproducibility Study: Design and Subjects

Reproducibility of the questionnaire was tested in 6 countries (Denmark, Norway, Iceland, Belgium, Portugal and Spain) according to the same protocol. The children filled in the questionnaire twice with an interval of 7–12 days. The reproducibility study was carried out in May to June 2003.

Subjects, 11-year-old boys and girls, were recruited through local schools and class teachers. Participation rates ranged between 78 and 100% [Denmark 82% (n = 62), Norway 86% (n = 71), Iceland 78% (n = 74), Belgium 92% (n = 66), Portugal 100% (n = 60), Spain 99% (n = 72)]. Age ranged between 11 and 12 years. The percentage of girls were: Denmark 69%, Norway 48%, Iceland 53%, Belgium 45%, Portugal 53%, Spain 39%.

Questionnaire

The dietary questionnaire includes two sections: a precoded 24-hour recall part asking in detail about yesterday's intake of fruit and vegetables and a food frequency part with 5 questions on usual intake of fruit and vegetables and 1 about intake of potatoes.

The first part of the questionnaire, the 24-hour recall section, was divided into 6 time intervals: morning/breakfast, midmorning, lunch, afternoon, evening meal, evening thereafter. Each interval started with a general question such as *'Did you eat or drink anything yesterday morning?'* (yes/no). *'What was it? (just write keywords as e.g. bread, milk, cornflakes, etc.)'*. These questions

Did you eat fruit yesterday morning? .... (write yes/no)

If yes,

What kind of fruit? How much?

(write 1 if you ate one apple, ½ if you ate a half)

Apple -------- **piece**

Banana -------- **piece**

Orange -------- **piece**

Tangerine -------- **piece**

Pear -------- **piece**

Melon -------- **piece**

Fruit salad -------- **piece**

Other fruit *(write which and how much)*

.... -------- **piece/portion**

.... -------- **piece/portion**

Fig. 1. An example of a precoded question on fruits in the 24-hour recall part.

Table 1. Portion sizes used for converting standard units into grams

Food item	24-hour recall g/portion or unit	Food frequency part g/times/day
Fruit		100
Apple, banana, orange, pear (pieces)	100	
Tangerine (piece)	50	
Melon (slice)	50	
Fruit salad (portion)[1]	50, 100, 150	
Other fruits (pieces/portion)	100	
Fruit juice	200	200
Raw vegetables		
Tomato (piece)	50	
Cucumber (slice)	10	
Carrot (piece)	65	
Other raw vegetables (portion)	50	50
Salad[1]	25, 50, 80, 130	40
Cooked vegetables[1]	40, 80, 150, 250	60

[1] The portion sizes in the photo series (see description of the 24-hour part of the questionnaire).

aimed at making the child think of actual intake on that specific day. After the general introductory question, the 24-hour recall section continued with questions on fruit and vegetable intake during each time interval (see examples in fig. 1). For each time interval, the participants were asked to record their intake of juice, fruit and raw vegetables, while salad, cooked vegetables and vegetable soup were only asked for lunch and evening meal. Amounts were indicated in terms of the number of *pieces, slices* or *portions* eaten, and standards were defined for these units (table 1). Three photo series were included in the questionnaire (for salad, for cooked vegetables and for fruit salad), each series showing three or four different portion sizes (table 1).

The second part of the dietary questionnaire, the food frequency section, included 5 questions about the usual frequency of intake for fresh fruit, salad, other raw vegetables, cooked vegetables and fruit juice. Also, in order to prevent misunderstanding, a separate question on potato intake was added to avoid that potatoes were included in the cooked vegetable answer. Eight response categories were used (never, less than 1 day/week, 1 day/week, 2–4 days/week, 5–6 days/week, every day, once/day, every day, twice/day, every day, more than twice/day). For the computation of frequencies into grams per day, see table 1. The participants were asked to think about their usual habits when filling in the food frequency part.

The questionnaire only includes fruit and vegetables eaten as such, whereas fruit and vegetables as part of composite dishes such as e.g. a stew of meat and vegetables or an apple pie, are not included.

The questionnaire was filled in by the children themselves in the classroom after the teacher had given a short instruction.

Pilot Tests

The development of the questionnaire included several pretests in schools, testing specific aspects (such as the format of the questions, the wording of the items, the number of precoded items listed, the portion size information and the layout). Different versions were tested and the level of understanding and the time needed to fill in were evaluated. The pretests were done in 4–7 of the participating Pro Children countries, with 50–120 children per country. One of the aspects investigated was the use of open-ended questions in the 24-hour recall section instead of precoded questions. The results showed that the open-ended version gave slightly lower mean intake than the precoded one, but that it required not only considerable additional coding work but also a number of interpretations that would be impossible to standardise across countries. Based on these results, it was decided to use the precoded version.

Food Records

Participants recorded their intake for 7 continuous days; the first day was a weighed record and the following 6 days were estimated records. The children and one of their parents were carefully instructed in how to keep the records, a written instruction was also handed out and a scale was provided for use on the first day. The first recording day was defined for each child by the researchers in order to achieve an even distribution of weighed food records between Mondays, Tuesdays, Wednesdays and Thursdays (the weekdays covered by the 24-hour recalls).

Only data on intake of fruit and vegetables were calculated from the food records. Data for intake of fruit and vegetable from the estimated records were converted from household units into grams in a similar way as for the 24-hour recall (table 1).

Table 2. Validity: Spearman correlation coefficients (r) of intakes (g/day) according to the food frequency questions and the reference method, 7-day food records

	Fruit	Total vegetables	Fruit and vegetables[1]	Orange juice
Denmark (n = 56)	0.47***	0.38**	0.46***	0.42**
Norway (n = 60)	0.46***	0.38**	0.45***	0.31*
Iceland (n = 43)	0.51***	0.53***	0.53***	0.55***
Portugal (n = 46)	0.43**	0.43**	0.40**	0.13

* $p < 0.05$; ** $p < 0.01$; *** $p < 0.001$.
[1] Not including orange juice intake.

Definitions

Only fresh fruits were defined as fruits. Potatoes were not included in the calculations of vegetable consumption. Vegetables and fruit as part of composite dishes were not included in the calculations. Total intake of fruit and vegetable was the sum of fruit and vegetables, excluding juice.

Data Analysis

The data were analysed using the SPSS statistical program version 11 (SPSS Inc., 1999). The validity of group mean intake from the 24-hour part was tested by comparison with results from the 1-day weighed food record. The validity and the reproducibility of the ranking of individuals according to the food frequency part were tested by comparison with results from the 7-day food record.

Differences between mean intakes were tested by paired t tests. Agreement between rankings was tested using Spearman rank correlation coefficients and by classification into intake quartiles.

Results

Validity

Table 2 shows Spearman rank correlations between intake of fruit and vegetable according to the food frequency part of the questionnaire and the reference method for that part, the 7-day food record. The correlations for total intake of fruit and vegetables ranged from 0.40 (Portugal) to 0.53 (Iceland). The correlations for fruit and vegetables separately were similar. For orange juice intake, the correlations ranged from 0.13 (Portugal) to 0.55 (Iceland). Cross-classification of subjects according to the food frequency and the 7-day food records is presented in table 3. Overall 25–50% were classified into the same quartile and 70–88% into the same or adjacent quartile. Between 0–12% were grossly misclassified into the opposite quartile.

Table 4 presents the intake of fruit and vegetables according to the 24-hour recall part of the questionnaire and the reference method for that part, the 1-day weighed food record. In Denmark, Norway and Iceland, no significant difference was observed for intake of fruit estimated with the two methods. For intake of vegetable, no significant difference was observed between the two methods in Denmark and Portugal, while a large difference was observed in Iceland and a smaller difference in Norway. For orange juice, significantly higher intakes were obtained with the 24-hour recall method in all 4 countries compared to the weighed record. Looking at the total intake of fruit and vegetables, no difference between the two methods was observed in Demark and Norway. In Iceland and Portugal, the 24-hour recall method gave significantly higher values for total intake of fruit and vegetables than the weighed record.

Table 3. Validity: Cross-classification of intake (g/day) into quartiles, according to the food frequency questions and the reference method, 7-day food records

	Percentage of subjects correctly classified into quartiles of intake		Grossly misclassified (opposite quartile)
	same quartile	same + adjacent quartile	
Denmark (n = 56)			
Fruit	39	78	5
Total vegetables	34	77	7
Fruit and vegetables[1]	50	80	2
Orange juice	25	77	0
Norway (n = 60)			
Fruit	48	80	3
Total vegetables	28	75	3
Fruit and vegetables[1]	42	77	3
Orange juice	38	73	12
Iceland (n = 43)			
Fruit	26	84	0
Total vegetables	35	88	2
Fruit and vegetables[1]	33	79	0
Orange juice	42	74	9
Portugal (n = 46)			
Fruit	37	70	7
Total vegetables	39	76	2
Fruit and vegetables[1]	39	78	2
Orange juice	32	73	0

[1] Not including orange juice intake.

Reproducibility

Reproducibility of the ranking of children according to their intake from the food frequency questions is presented in tables 5 and 6. In general, the correlations between intake from the first and the second round were

Table 4. Intake (g/day) according to the 24-hour recall results and the reference method, 1-day weighed food record (WFR_{1d})

	24-hour recall	WFR_{1d}	Difference	p value
Denmark (n = 56)				
Fruit	147 (0, 200)	155 (0, 275)	–8	0.72
Total vegetables	106 (25, 140)	84 (12, 141)	22	0.17
Fruit and vegetables[1]	253 (100, 360)	239 (115, 375)	14	0.59
Orange juice	158 (0, 300)	36 (0, 0)	122	<0.0001
Norway (n = 60)				
Fruit	140 (13, 200)	140 (0, 215)	0	0.98
Total vegetables	84 (0, 118)	50 (0, 76)	34	0.043
Fruit and vegetables[1]	224 (91, 318)	190 (54, 270)	34	0.25
Orange juice	160 (0, 200)	75 (0, 168)	85	0.012
Iceland (n = 43)				
Fruit	160 (75, 250)	121 (0, 220)	39	0.068
Total vegetables	82 (0, 115)	17 (0, 0)	65	0.001
Fruit and vegetables[1]	242 (100, 360)	138 (0, 231)	104	0.001
Orange juice	267 (0, 400)	40 (0, 0)	227	0.000
Portugal (n = 46)				
Fruit	189 (100, 300)	122 (0, 182)	67	0.004
Total vegetables	60 (0, 81)	42 (0, 75)	18	0.212
Fruit and vegetables[1]	249 (119, 345)	164 (29, 258)	85	0.006
Orange juice	83 (0, 200)	19 (0, 0)	65	0.002

Results are means, with the 25th percentile and 75th percentile in parentheses.
[1] Not including orange juice intake.

high, ranging between 0.47 and 0.84, with averages of 0.65 for fruit, 0.67 for vegetables, 0.69 for the total intake of fruit and vegetables and 0.72 for orange juice (table 5). However, small variations between countries were observed.

Cross-classification of subjects according to the first and the second round showed that between 39 and 72% were placed in the same quartile and 85–98% in the same or adjacent quartile (table 6). Between 0 and 8% were grossly misclassified into the opposite quartile.

Table 5. Reproducibility: Spearman correlation coefficients (r) of intakes (g/day) from food frequency questions according to the first and the second round

	Fruit	Total vegetable	Fruit and vegetable[1]	Orange juice
Denmark (n = 62)	0.47	0.71	0.58	0.81
Norway (n = 71)	0.67	0.66	0.68	0.67
Iceland (n = 74)	0.76	0.66	0.71	0.56
Belgium (n = 66)	0.69	0.64	0.72	0.71
Portugal (n = 60)	0.56	0.59	0.74	0.73
Spain (n = 72)	0.77	0.74	0.69	0.84

All correlations were significant, $p < 0.001$.
[1] Not including orange juice intake.

Discussion

Measuring food intake is a challenge in all age groups, but perhaps particularly challenging among children, especially when parents are not involved. In the present study, the validity and the reproducibility of a dietary questionnaire for measuring intake of fruit and vegetables were investigated in several European countries according to the same protocol. The validation study showed a fairly good ranking of the children according to their intake of fruit and vegetables, based on the food frequency part, in all 4 countries. Moreover, the results showed that the 24-hour recall part gave valid estimates for average intake of fruit in 3 of the 4 countries and valid average intake of vegetables in 2 countries. However, in Iceland and in Norway, the 24-hour recall part overestimated intake of vegetables compared to the reference method, while this was the case for fruit in Portugal.

A number of validation studies of fruit and vegetable questionnaires have been published [16], however, only few focused on children [8–10, 12, 15, 17]. The observed

Table 6. Reproducibility: Cross-classification of intake according to the food frequency questions (g/day) in the first and the second round

	Percentage of subjects correctly classified into quartiles of intake		Grossly mis-classified (opposite quartile)
	same quartile	same + adjacent quartile	
Denmark (n = 62)			
Fruit	56	85	8
Total vegetables	55	90	2
Fruit and vegetables[1]	42	89	5
Orange juice	60	94	0
Norway (n = 71)			
Fruit	52	90	0
Total vegetables	39	90	3
Fruit and vegetables[1]	44	87	4
Orange juice	56	86	3
Iceland (n = 74)			
Fruit	47	89	0
Total vegetables	51	86	0
Fruit and vegetables[1]	53	88	4
Orange juice	43	93	4
Belgium (n = 66)			
Fruit	56	89	0
Total vegetables	50	86	0
Fruit and vegetables[1]	52	91	3
Orange juice	53	92	2
Portugal (n = 60)			
Fruit	55	88	3
Total vegetables	48	85	5
Fruit and vegetables[1]	50	75	2
Orange juice	72	92	3
Spain (n = 72)			
Fruit	58	96	0
Total vegetables	47	89	0
Fruit and vegetables[1]	56	87	3
Orange juice	51	98	0

[1] Not including orange juice intake.

correlation coefficients between fruit and vegetable intake estimated with the food frequency part and the 7-day food record reference method are similar to or even higher than what other researchers have reported for fruit and vegetables measured by frequency questions among children and adolescents [8–10, 12, 15, 16]. These results indicate that the 11-year-old children are able to give fairly valid and consistent information about their frequency of intake of fruit and vegetables.

The observed tendency to a somewhat higher mean intake obtained with the 24-hour recall part of the questionnaire compared to the food record has previously been reported by Andersen et al. [8] among 12-year-old children and by Eriksen et al. [15] among 6- to 10-year-olds. In these studies, the questionnaire was administered in a different way than in the present study; in the study by Andersen et al. [8] by reading the questions out loud to the class, one by one, and in the study by Eriksen et al. [15] the questionnaire was filled in at home with the possibility of help from the parents.

The validity of the questionnaire was tested in 4 countries, 2 Nordic countries where national intake of fruit and vegetable is moderate (Denmark and Norway), 1 Nordic country with a low national intake (Iceland) and 1 southern European country where national intake is relatively high (Portugal). Similar validity and reproducibility results were obtained in all 4 countries with respect to ranking of the children, whereas the validity of the mean intake assessment was better in Norway and Denmark than in Portugal and Iceland where we found strong indications that either fruit intake (Portugal) or vegetable intake (Iceland) was significantly overestimated in the 24-hour recall part. It may be that the children tended to overreport intake in the 24-hour part because they were aware that fruit and vegetable are healthy and gave socially desirable answers, and that this tendency was more pronounced in 2 of the countries. However, if that was the case, the same tendency would be expected in the food frequency part, and comparisons of mean intakes obtained from the food frequency part and the food records did not indicate such overestimations. Differences in reading and understanding capabilities at the age of 11 between different countries may also play a role. Further analyses of the validity results indicated that the overestimation problems encountered with the 24-hour part of the questionnaire in the 2 countries were related to two aspects: the division of the day into 6 time intervals and the photos used for portion estimation. For example, many children in Denmark and Portugal reported exactly the same consumption of fruit or vegetable 'at lunch' and 'in the afternoon', indicating that the same consumption was reported twice. Thus, the results indicated that it would be an advantage to divide the day into fewer time intervals in order to avoid that some children repeated exactly the same food item and quantity on two or more occasions without realising that they were reporting one eating occasion twice. Also, the validity study results showed that the photos used for individual estimation of portion sizes (for salad, cooked vegetables and fruit salad/berries; see Methods) sometimes caused considerable confusion and obvious errors; for example some children were ticking off relatively large photo portions of several foods in the same time interval. This indicates that in this age group photos can only be used if considerably more time is available for explaining their use (as had been the case in the pretests preceding the validity study).

Based on these results of the validity study, it was decided to modify the 24-hour section of the questionnaire so that the day was divided into only 3 periods (morning and midmorning, lunch and afternoon, evening meal and evening) instead of 6, and the photos were left out and substituted by standard portions. These adjustments were included in the final version of the questionnaire used in the Pro Children study.

In the reproducibility study, the correlation coefficients between intakes according to the food frequency part filled in at time 1 (test) and time 2 (retest) were high for all 6 countries involved. Similar results were observed for the children in the studies by Eriksen et al. [15] and Andersen et al. [8]. The good reproducibility results indicate that the children are able to report their frequency of intake of fruit and vegetable in a consistent way.

Conclusions

The validity of the questionnaire was satisfactory as to ranking children according to their usual intake of fruit and vegetables, based on the food frequency part of the questionnaire. This ranking is a key aspect in this project since it is a necessary prerequisite for investigating potential determinants of intake. The validity of the group mean intake, based on the original 24-hour part of the questionnaire, was satisfactory for fruit in 3 of the 4 countries and for vegetables in 2 of the countries. The 24-hour part was subsequently adjusted, in order to avoid overestimation of intake, by reducing the number of time intervals during the day, and by leaving out the photos for portion size estimation of certain vegetables and fruit which were included in the original version. The two sections of the questionnaire, the frequency part and the 24-hour part, complement each other, and the adjusted questionnaire is used in the Pro Children Project to investigate determinants of intake and fruit and vegetable intervention effects in European schoolchildren.

Acknowledgement

This study is being carried out with financial support from the Commission of the European Communities, specific RTD programme 'Quality of Life and Management of Living Resources', QLK1-2001-00547 'Promoting and Sustaining Health through Increased Fruit and Vegetable Consumption among European Schoolchildren' (Pro Children). The study does not necessarily reflect the Commission's views and in no way anticipates the Commission's future policy in this area.

References

1 Andersen LF, Overby N, Lillegaard IT: Intake of fruit and vegetables among Norwegian children and adolescents (in Norwegian). Tidsskr Nor Laegeforen 2004;124:1396–1398.

2 Pomerleau J, Lock K, McKee M, Altmann DR: The challenge of measuring global fruit and vegetable intake. J Nutr 2004;134:1175–1180.

3 Cavadini C, Siega-Riz AM, Popkin BM: US adolescent food intake trends from 1965 to 1996. West J Med 2000;173:378–383.

4 Klepp K-I, Pérez-Rodrigo C, De Bourdeaudhuij I, Due P, Elmadfa I, Haraldsdóttir J, König J, Sjöström M, Thórsdóttir I, de Almeida MDV, Yngve A, Brug J: Promoting fruit and vegetable consumption among European schoolchildren: rationale, conceptualization and design of the Pro Children Project. Ann Nutr Metab 2005;49;212–220.

5 Hammond J, Nelson M, Chinn S, Rona RJ: Validation of a food frequency questionnaire for assessing dietary intake in a study of coronary heart disease risk factors in children. Eur J Clin Nutr 1993;47:242–250.

6 Livingstone MB, Robson PJ: Measurement of dietary intake in children. Proc Nutr Soc 2000; 59:279–293.

7 Baranowski T, Domel SB: A cognitive model of children's reporting of food intake. Am J Clin Nutr 1994;59:212S–217S.

8 Andersen LF, Bere E, Kolbjornsen N, Klepp KI: Validity and reproducibility of self-reported intake of fruit and vegetable among 6th graders. Eur J Clin Nutr 2004;58:771–777.

9 Baranowski T, Smith M, Baranowski J, Wang DT, Doyle C, Lin LS, Hearn MD, Resnicow K: Low validity of a seven-item fruit and vegetable food frequency questionnaire among third-grade students. J Am Diet Assoc 1997;97:66–68.

10 Domel SB, Baranowski T, Davis H, Leonard SB, Riley P, Baranowski J: Fruit and vegetable food frequency by fourth and fifth grade students: validity and reliability. J Am Coll Nutr 1994;13:33–39.

11 Edmunds LD, Ziebland S: Development and validation of the Day in the Life Questionnaire (DILQ) as a measure of fruit and vegetable questionnaire for 7- to 9-year-olds. Health Educ Res 2002;17:211–220.

12 Field AE, Peterson KE, Gortmaker SL, Cheung L, Rockett H, Fox MK, Colditz GA: Reproducibility and validity of a food frequency questionnaire among fourth to seventh grade inner-city school children: implication of age and day-to-day variation in dietary intake. Public Health Nutr 1999;2:293–300.

13 Lytle LA, Murray DM, Perry CL, Eldridge AL: Validating fourth-grade students' self-report of dietary intake: results from the 5 A Day Power Plus program. J Am Diet Assoc 1998;98:570–572.

14 Vereecken CA, Maes L: A Belgian study on the reliability and relative validity of the Health Behaviour in School-Aged Children food-frequency questionnaire. Public Health Nutr 2003;6:581–588.

15 Eriksen K, Haraldsdottir J, Pederson R, Flyger HV: Effect of a fruit and vegetable subscription in Danish schools. Public Health Nutr 2003;6: 57–63.

16 van Assema P, Brug J, Ronda G, Steenhuis I, Oenema A: A short Dutch questionnaire to measure fruit and vegetable intake: relative validity among adults and adolescents. Nutr Health 2002;16:85–106.

17 Field AE, Colditz GA, Fox MK, Byers T, Serdula M, Bosch RJ, Peterson KE: Comparison of 4 questionnaires assessment of fruit and vegetable intake. Am J Public Health 1998;88: 1216–1218.

Annals of
Nutrition & Metabolism

Ann Nutr Metab 2005;49:228–235
DOI: 10.1159/000087246

Published online: July 28, 2005

A Qualitative Exploration of Determinants of Fruit and Vegetable Intake among 10- and 11-Year-Old Schoolchildren in the Low Countries

Marianne Wind[a] Kelly Bobelijn[b] Ilse De Bourdeaudhuij[b] Knut-Inge Klepp[c]
Johannes Brug[a]

[a]Department of Public Health, Erasmus MC, University Medical Center Rotterdam, Rotterdam, The Netherlands;
[b]Department of Movement and Sports Sciences, Ghent University, Ghent, Belgium; [c]Department of Nutrition, Faculty of Medicine, University of Oslo, Oslo, Norway

Key Words
Focus groups · European schoolchildren · Determinants of fruit and vegetable intake

Abstract
Background: For the development of fruit and vegetable promotion interventions, insight is needed into determinants of health behaviour. This study presents results of focus group interviews held with 10- to 11-year-old schoolchildren from Ghent (Belgium-Flanders) and Rotterdam (the Netherlands) to explore personal beliefs and motivations and environmental factors related to schoolchildren's fruit and vegetable intake, to inform the Pro Children intervention development. ***Methods:*** Twelve focus groups were held with 92 schoolchildren. The interviews were recorded and transcribed and NVivo was used to analyse the transcripts. ***Results:*** Positive health beliefs, taste preferences, lack of knowledge and practical barriers were identified as personal factors related to fruit and vegetable intake. Home and school availability of fruits and vegetables, as well as parenting practices were identified as important environmental factors. ***Conclusion:*** A fruit and vegetable promotion intervention should aim to increase fruit and vegetable accessibility and should include educational and motivational activities tailored to these personal and environmental factors. These indications should be further evaluated in quantitative research among representative samples.

K.-I.K. and J.B. designed this study. M.W. and K.B. conducted the focus groups and M.W. analysed the transcripts under supervision of J.B. and I.B.; M.W. wrote the first draft of the paper, which was revised by J.B.; K.B., K.-I.K. and I.B. commented on this second draft and M.W. then wrote the final draft of the present paper.

Background

The 'Pro Children' study aims to systematically develop and test evidence- and theory-based strategies to promote adequate consumption levels of fruit and vegetable among primary schoolchildren across Europe [1]. Intervention development and evaluation of the Pro Children study was therefore informed by the Intervention Mapping protocol [2]. According to Intervention Mapping as well as other health promotion planning models like the Precede-Proceed model [3], a first essential step in intervention development is to gain insight into important and changeable determinants of the target behaviour. Such knowledge about behavioural determi-

KARGER
Fax +41 61 306 12 34
E-Mail karger@karger.ch
www.karger.com

© 2005 S. Karger AG, Basel
0250–6807/05/0494–0228$22.00/0

Accessible online at:
www.karger.com/anm

Marianne Wind
Department of Public Health, Erasmus MC
University Medical Centre Rotterdam, PO Box 1738
NL–3000 DR Rotterdam (The Netherlands)
Tel. +31 10 408 82 69/77 14, Fax +31 10 408 94 49, E-Mail m.wind@erasmusmc.nl

nants helps to identify specific learning and performance objectives for the intervention, and interventions should be tailored to these determinants to improve the chance for effects [2, 3]. To explore and describe determinants of health behaviour, several methods are appropriate, such as problem-driven and theory-driven literature searches and original qualitative and quantitative research [2]. If a certain issue has already extensively been researched, exploring the relevant literature may be sufficient to identify the most relevant determinants. However, hardly any studies on important and changeable determinants of fruit and vegetable intake in 10- to 11-year-old children have been conducted in most European countries, including Belgium and the Netherlands [4–9]. In such cases, explorative, qualitative methods are most appropriate to start a determinants study. An example of a useful qualitative research method is the focus group interview, which is an effective technique to investigate eating behaviour [10–12].

We applied focus group interviews among 5th- and 6th-grade primary schoolchildren in Ghent (Belgium-Flanders) and Rotterdam (the Netherlands) as part of the stepwise development of the Pro Children Project. The purpose of this study was to identify personal beliefs and motivations as well as possible environmental factors that are related to schoolchildren's fruit and vegetable intake. Special attention was given to differences in potential determinants according to gender, ethnicity and country.

Method

A focus group is a small group of people who, led by a moderator, discuss several topics concerning a specific subject in which a research team is interested. To ensure that all participants will join in, the group should not be larger than 8–10 participants [13, 14]. When younger children are involved, groups should preferably be somewhat smaller, since children may be less familiar with expressing their opinion in a group setting. The moderator's task is to encourage the exchange of ideas and opinions, to ensure that the interview discussions stay focused on the interview topic, but to intervene as little as possible [13, 14]. As suggested by Morgan and Krueger [13] and others [11, 14–16], we composed an interview guide to facilitate the focus groups. Development of the guide was based on findings from literature reviews [17] and recent original qualitative studies [10–12] investigating determinants of schoolchildren's fruit and vegetable intake in countries outside Europe. The guide was reviewed by different experts on nutrition and health education from the Pro Children consortium and further enriched based on their comments.

Ethical approval for the Pro Children study was obtained from medical ethical committees in both countries, and schools provided informed consent and full cooperation.

Before the start of the interviews, the children were told that their names would remain anonymous.

During the interviews, questions to explore determinants of fruit and vegetable consumption were asked separately, since it was expected that schoolchildren, in line with adults [18], may have different motivations for eating fruit and vegetable. Many psychosocial theories, such as the Health Belief Model and the Theory of Planned Behaviour (see for example Glanz et al. [19] and Conner and Norman [20] for good overviews) are often applied to investigate health behaviour and the individual behavioural determinants, such as attitudes, subjective norms, perceived control, personal risk perceptions and motivation to change behaviour. Recently, more attention has been paid to social ecological models that emphasize the importance of ecological determinants (i.e. the physical or social environment) [21].

Earlier research indicated that personal factors may account for only a small percentage of the variability in children's fruit and vegetable intake [17] and several studies have shown the importance of environmental determinants in shaping eating habits of schoolchildren [5, 22, 23]. Therefore, possible personal factors (such as attitudes, outcome expectations, perceived barriers, taste preferences, estimation of own intake, skills and knowledge), as well as possible environmental factors (such as availability and accessibility, peer and parental influences) were discussed during the interviews. Because eating behaviour is complex and difficult to explain and change, Baranowski et al. [17, 24] suggested to explain situational fruit and vegetable intake, and not fruit and vegetable intake in general. Because schoolchildren spend a large proportion of the day at school and at home, we included separate questions to identify personal and environmental factors of fruit and vegetable intake in the school and home situation.

Participants

Twelve focus group interviews were conducted with a total of 92 schoolchildren living in Belgium-Flanders or the Netherlands. In both countries, a convenient sample of schools was selected. In *the Netherlands,* 8 focus group interviews were carried out at 3 different schools in the city of Rotterdam. In total, 60 schoolchildren were interviewed (29 boys and 31 girls). Of the eight groups, two groups consisted only of boys, one only of girls and the remaining groups were of mixed gender. Most groups consisted of 7 or 8 schoolchildren (range 5–10 children) and all were 10 or 11 years old. Reflecting the cultural diversity of the inhabitants of Rotterdam, almost all schoolchildren who participated in the first 5 interviews were from cultural and ethnic minority groups and had at least one parent who was born in a foreign country (i.e. Turkey, Morocco, Surinam, Pakistan, Yugoslavia, Bosnia, the Netherlands Antilles, the Dominican Republic and Ghana). For this reason, 3 more focus group interviews were conducted at a third school. With the exception of one child, all the children at this school had both parents born in the Netherlands.

In *Belgium-Flanders,* 4 focus group interviews were performed in the city of Ghent. In total, 32 schoolchildren took part in the interviews (16 boys and 16 girls). One group consisted only of boys, one only of girls and the remaining groups were of mixed gender. All groups consisted of 8 schoolchildren and all were 10 or 11 years old. Only 4 schoolchildren had parents born in a foreign country (i.e. Spain, Turkey and Morocco). Both in Belgium-Flanders and the Netherlands, all schoolchildren were fifth and sixth graders.

Procedure

Because of small differences in language and dialect between Belgium-Flanders and the Netherlands, a native speaker researcher led the interviews in each country. In both countries, an assistant was present to take notes, to notice non-verbal behaviour during the interviews and to monitor the process. To make the schoolchildren feel more comfortable, they first had to introduce themselves and name their favourite kind of fruit and vegetable. After discussing all possible determinants of schoolchildren's fruit and vegetable intake, a piece of fruit and a can of fruit juice were handed out to the schoolchildren as a reward for participation. Each interview took about 45–60 min and was tape-recorded.

Analyses

After each interview, the moderator and assistant discussed the interview and relevant non-verbal behaviour. After all the interviews had been conducted, transcripts were made. M.W. did the first analyses of the transcripts using NVivo version 1.3 [25]. Possible determinants were analysed separately for fruit and vegetable intake. For both fruit and vegetable intake, a further initial distinction was made between personal factors, factors related to the school environment and factors related to the home environment. This distinction was based on the literature study that formed the basis for the interview guide. Furthermore, during analyses special attention was given to differences in potential determinants according to gender, ethnicity or country. K.B. did a secondary analysis of all transcripts and results. If the researchers had made different interpretations, J.B. was asked to judge the data and the interpretation was discussed until consensus was reached.

Results

The results are presented according to the aforementioned distinction between personal and environmental determinants. In the description of the results, we include quotes from the interviews in parentheses to illustrate certain factors.

Personal Factors

Health Beliefs

Expecting positive health outcomes from, or prescribing positive attributes to eating fruit and vegetable was mentioned most often as a reason to eat fruit and vegetable. Most participants knew fruit and vegetable are healthy and contain vitamins, and they are supposed to 'make you strong' ('I eat fruit and vegetable because it is good for your body. It contains vitamin C.').

Taste Preferences

Besides health aspects, taste preferences were often mentioned as a factor related to eating fruit and vegetable. Many participants said they did (not) eat fruit and vegetable simply because they (did not) like them. Most participants seemed to prefer fruit to vegetables. Some vegetables were considered too bitter ('I don't like vegetables, they are often too bitter. Only grown-up's like that.'). Vegetable juices were also less popular than fruit juices, because they were considered less tasty. Only a few participants said they sometimes drunk tomato juice or carrot juice, while fruit juices were very popular among the participants.

Knowledge

To assess knowledge of fruit and vegetable, we asked participants to mention examples of fruit, fruit juices and vegetables. It seemed that children from ethnic minorities were more familiar with 'exotic' fruits and vegetables like mango, pineapple or squash.

Knowledge about fruit juices was often incorrect, especially in the Netherlands. Several of the participants thought that all kinds of soft drinks, lemonades, fruit yoghurt, milk shakes or even fruit tea could be defined as fruit juice.

We also asked whether children were familiar with the national guidelines for recommended intake. Dutch participants seemed to be more aware of the recommended intake for fruit compared to the Flemish participants. In both Belgium-Flanders and the Netherlands, most participants were not familiar with national guidelines for vegetable intake ('I think two tablespoons of vegetables each day is enough.').

Awareness

When asking participants whether they thought they ate enough fruit and vegetable themselves, almost all participants thought they did. However, when asking them whether they ate fruit and vegetable every day, hardly anybody actually said that they did so.

Personal Barriers

Several personal barriers were mentioned. Many participants said it was not common to eat fruit and vegetable during leisure time activities, because they forgot to take them with them, they just wanted to play, or they were too busy to remember to eat fruit ('My mother often forgets to put fruit in my bag, sometimes I remember. But I often forget to do that too'.). Fruit getting squashed in the (school) bag was also mentioned as a reason for not eating fruit ('I don't take fruit with me in my bag. I throw my bag around and then it gets squashed.'). Participants seemed to be quite choosy when it comes to eating fruit. Besides taste, the appearance of fruit was considered important. Some participants said they did not want to eat fruit when, for example, it contained seeds, when it was too hard, too sweet, too sour or too bitter ('When I eat an apple, I only eat the middle of it, I do not like the peel.'). Finally, many participants mentioned that sweets were competitors for eating fruit and vegetable ('I am allowed to take candies or cookies with me. I prefer those.').

Factors Related to the School Environment

Availability

About half of the participants ate lunch at school; the other half went home for lunch, at least on most school days. In the Flemish schools, children could get soup and/or a hot meal at school, whereas in the Netherlands this was uncommon. School food was usually not available at Dutch schools. Dutch children who stayed at school during the lunch break had to bring their lunches from home. Although in both countries parents often prepared their children's lunchboxes, most children also had a say when it comes to preparing the lunch. In both countries, many children said they usually did not take fruit with them to school; bringing vegetables to school was even less common.

Peer Influences

Although many participants seemed to be convinced that other children did not influence their fruit and vegetable intake, some indirect influence by peers could be detected. Peer influence may be especially strong on behaviours that may compete with fruit and vegetable intake, such as eating candies ('I do feel like eating candy when I see somebody eating sweets, but I do not feel the urge to eat an apple when I see somebody eating an apple.').

Social Norms

Eating fruit at school was perceived as 'normal' by most children. Participants who did not eat fruit at school themselves did not find it strange that other children ate fruit at school. Only when it comes to birthdays or other celebrations, social norms tended to steer children away from eating fruit ('When it is somebody's birthday, you do not serve fruit.'; 'Nobody likes that, children want to eat candy when it is a party.'). Serving vegetables was considered to be a rather unusual and certainly not a preferred thing to do at such occasions ('You eat vegetables during dinner, not at school.'). However, among participants from minority groups, it seemed to be more common to eat raw vegetables during school hours ('Sometimes my mother prepares a sandwich with lettuce and tomato for me to take to school.').

School Food Policies

Most participating children were not aware of school food policies, such as rules about foods that cannot be used for birthday treats at school. When school food policies were known, the children indicated that neither they nor their parents complied with these rules. Influences from teachers were perceived as marginal. According to the participating children, their teachers rarely encouraged them to eat fruit and vegetable during breaks or when celebrating birthdays.

Factors Related to the Home Environment

Family Influences

Children reported that their parents seemed to have a lot of influence on their fruit and vegetable intake. According to the participants, their parents often decided whether and what vegetables would be served for dinner and what their child would eat at school ('At my father's place, we just have to eat what he prepares.').

Children shared the opinion that their parents were responsible for buying fruits and vegetables. But, according to most participants, the parents took into account their preference when purchasing fruits and vegetables.

Some children went shopping themselves instead of asking for the kind of fruits or vegetables they wanted. When children went shopping on their own, they did not use their pocket money, since that was reserved for sweets, games and such.

These interviews gave the impression that children from minority groups went shopping on their own more often and seemed to be more inclined to buy fruit themselves ('When I feel like eating grapes, I just go to the supermarket myself.'). Nevertheless, most of these children also preferred to spend their money for other purposes than eating fruit or vegetables.

Availability and Accessibility

Dutch participants reported that vegetables were often not available at home, whereas according to the Flemish participants vegetables were often available. Fruit seemed to be unavailable during part of the week both in the Netherlands and in Belgium-Flanders ('Every Saturday my parents go to the market, so on Friday sometimes there is no fruit left.'). When fruit was available at home, it was often stored in a visible place such as on a fruit bowl on the table. According to participants from ethnic minorities, it was more common to put a fruit bowl on the table when other family members were visiting them.

Most Dutch participants were allowed to take fruit themselves whenever they wanted. Only when participants tended to eat 'too much fruit', parents sometimes interfered. In Belgium-Flanders, participants more often had to ask whether they could take fruit ('When I am at my father's place I have to ask, when I am at my mother's I can just take it myself.'). Taking and eating vegetables without asking was uncommon for participants in both countries.

Vegetables were typically eaten at dinner in both the Netherlands and Belgium-Flanders where it is common to eat one hot meal per day that traditionally includes vegetables [26]. Therefore, not having vegetables for dinner was often mentioned as an important reason for not eating vegetables during that day.

Eating vegetables during other meals or in between meals seemed to be quite unusual. Only a few participants, mainly from minority groups, said they sometimes ate a piece of cucumber, carrot or a tomato as a snack in between meals.

Eating fruit throughout the day was more common ('I eat fruit when I feel like it.'). Nevertheless, most participants did not eat fruit at school, but rather at home after school, since they did not want to take fruit to school because it tends to get squashed in the schoolbag. Orange juice typically belonged to breakfast according to some participants, and is thus not something to drink during the rest of the day ('Every morning I drink a glass of orange juice. That always is part of my breakfast.').

Some participants said they more often ate fruit during the weekends than on school days, because they had more time and there was more fresh fruit available at home than at school. Others ate less fruit over the weekends because they were too busy doing other things and did not remember to eat fruit.

Vegetables were less often part of the dinner during weekends, because it was more common to eat take-away food or eat out then ('During the week we eat something like broccoli, but during the weekend we eat French fries.').

Food Rules

Since many of the participants appreciated vegetables less than fruit, some parents applied rules, such as demanding that their child eat some vegetables. However, the children often got away with it, because several participants reported that they were allowed to dish up their own vegetables and would take small helpings ('I have to eat all my veggies, but I can dish up my own plate. It doesn't matter how much I take.'). A few participants mentioned they had to at least taste the vegetables. In some families, children were punished when not eating their vegetables (e.g. no dessert, no television) or they got rewarded when finishing them. This seemed to stimulate the participants to finish their dinner ('When we eat something I don't like, I have to finish it, otherwise I am not allowed to leave the table. So I finish my plate.').

Encouragement

According to the participating children, some parents actively encouraged them to eat fruit and vegetable, either by saying they have to eat fruit and vegetable or by preparing fruit as a snack and vegetables for dinner ('My mother says it is healthy.'). Eating vegetables in between meals was more unusual than eating fruit as a snack, and therefore parents seemed to pay less attention to eating vegetables. However, many participants did not experience parental encouragement to eat fruit either.

Especially when participants do not like fruit, it seemed fruit should be made as accessible as possible ('When my mother does not tell me, it sometimes happens that I do not eat fruit for a week.').

In Belgium-Flanders, participants said they were often not allowed to cut vegetables themselves or to help preparing dinner, but they could prepare fruit (e.g. fruit salad, fruit shake). In the Netherlands, on the other hand, many participants were allowed to and liked to prepare fruit as well as vegetable dishes. The participants especially liked to prepare fruit salads or mixed fruit juices, desserts or fruit cake. The Dutch interviews also gave the impression that participants from minorities prepared dinner themselves more often.

Discussion

The results from this study suggest the relevance of personal determinants related to schoolchildren's fruit and vegetable intake. Taste preferences for specific kinds of fruit and vegetable and having a positive health belief related to eating fruit and vegetable were mentioned most often. Other personal factors that seem to influence intake were perceived barriers, i.e. forgetting to eat fruit and vegetable, a stronger preference for competing foods such as sweets, being choosy when it comes to fruit and inadequate knowledge of recommended intake levels. Not knowing the recommended intake levels might lead to an overestimation of own fruit and vegetable intake. Although we conducted part of our focus group interviews in separate gender groups, we did not uncover indications of strong differences in determinants between boys and girls.

From quantitative studies it is known that many children aged 10–13 years do not meet the recommendations for fruit and vegetable intake [27], while other studies have shown that adolescents [28] as well as adults [29] overestimate the adequacy of their intake levels. Our study provides some indication that this also applies to younger children.

In both the school and home environment, availability of fruit and vegetable seems to influence intake of these foods by schoolchildren. At Belgian-Flemish and Dutch primary schools, there is no or hardly any food available. In Belgium-Flanders, fruit is available only in 14% of the primary schools [30]. In both countries, most schoolchildren who eat lunch at school bring their own lunchbox that is often prepared by their parents. Yet, parents seem to take their child's preferences into account when preparing their lunchbox. Unfortunately, parents often forget to give their child fruit or vegetables when going to school, or the schoolchildren themselves prefer to take other food with them.

Children do not seem to be aware of any enforced school food policies. They are allowed to bring other food items, such as cakes, cookies, bread or candies with them to school; because of this, many participants do not eat fruit at school. In the Netherlands, formulating a school health policy is obligatory, but the school itself can determine the content of the policy by deciding which health topics will be addressed [31]. In Belgium-Flanders, most primary schools have written rules, but only to restrict intake of savoury snacks and sweet snacks [30].

At school, social norms and peer influences only seem to play a role when treats are provided at birthdays. Based on what the children say, in this age group parents influence schoolchildren's intake of fruit and vegetable more than peers do. Parents are often responsible for buying and preparing fruit and vegetable and for making them more available and accessible at home. In some families, parents are also quite active in encouraging their children to eat fruit and vegetable by preparing these for their children or by applying food rules.

Preferences, health beliefs and home and parental practices were also identified as the major influences in earlier qualitative and quantitative studies. Baranowski et al. [11] identified home availability and affect as major influences on fruit and vegetable intake. In that study, affect was described as combining two factors: preferences and expectancies (knowing that it is good for you). Baranowski et al. [11] identified skills as a third main determinant. In our study, we did not obtain detailed information on specific skills, such as asking parents to buy or prepare special kinds of fruits and vegetables. However, the interviews did indicate that 'asking skills' could be a relevant factor for children in order to encourage their parents to make fruits and vegetables more readily available. Bauer et al. [12] also indicated the importance of addressing environmental factors to promote healthy eating habits in adolescents.

Focus groups enable the collection of extensive and valuable information in a relatively short period of time. Group interactions and observing non-verbal communication helps researchers to stimulate discussions and to uncover in-depth data [13]. However, focus groups do not provide hard evidence on the relative importance of potential behavioural determinants, nor do they provide a representative picture of important behavioural influences. Furthermore, some children may not be used to such discussions and dominant or shy children could hinder the process of the focus groups or bias the outcomes [14].

Nevertheless, qualitative data as derived from focus groups can provide useful information when designing a school-based intervention. Asking schoolchildren themselves to describe their views and thoughts in their own words enables intervention developers to target the intervention to the needs of schoolchildren. Young people's views should be the starting point for any future efforts to promote healthy eating [32].

Due to small language differences between Belgium-Flanders and the Netherlands, two moderators guided the interviews. Differences in experience and interviewing style may have affected the flow and content of the interviews [15]. However, both moderators communicated regularly and used a well-structured interview guide. Although this interview guide may have reduced a possible moderator bias, it also somewhat restricted the openness of the discussion among the children, which may have prevented more unexpected determinants from being detected. However, focus groups are most effective when these are at least somewhat structured and when specific questions are formulated [11, 13, 16]. We conducted a standard analysis procedure, with one researcher doing the primary analyses and a second researcher doing the checking of transcripts and a second analysis, in order to optimise the reliability and validity of the outcomes [15, 16].

As a consequence of selecting schools at random in only two cities, the results of this study might not be generally representative. Fruit and vegetable intake between boys and girls does differ [27, 33]; however, we did not uncover strong differences in potential determinants between boys and girls. We found only small differences between participants from both countries and ethnic minority groups. Therefore, quantitative survey research, preferably with a longitudinal design, as well as evaluations of interventions that address these factors are needed to further verify the relationship between the personal and environmental determinants we explored and schoolchildren's fruit and vegetable intake [17]. Such research methods would allow more solid conclusions to be drawn regarding differences in determinants according to gender, ethnicity or country. This is indeed what is being carried out within the Pro Children study, with a cross-sectional cross-national survey among more than 13,000 European schoolchildren and their parents and intervention studies in 3 European countries [1]. To conduct such a quantitative study and to evaluate effects of the intervention, valid and reliable assessment instruments are crucial. The results of this study have therefore also been used as input for the development of a questionnaire to assess schoolchildren's fruit and vegetable intake and its determinants [34].

To increase the likelihood of behaviour change, an intervention should be tailored to mediators [17, 24]. Nowadays, the health promotion literature emphasizes the inclusion of environmental changes in interventions in order to make 'the healthy choice, the easy choice', especially related to obesity prevention [35] and fruit and vegetable intake in youth [36]. Our findings indicate the need to design an intervention that is tailored to personal as well as environmental determinants. Similar to other studies, our study also showed that taste preferences [5, 37] and increasing availability in the home [23, 37] are important determinants that should be addressed.

The present study indicates that fruit and vegetable promotion in children should focus on improving availability of fruits and vegetables and on improving fruit- and vegetable-related health beliefs and preferences. To improve home availability parents should be involved since they have primary responsibility for buying and preparing fruit and vegetable. This could either be done directly by means of an intervention or indirectly by teaching children specific asking skills. Baranowski et al. [24] suggest developing separate interventions aimed at behaviour change in separate situations. The present study suggests that vegetable promotion for 10- to 11-year-old children in the Low Countries should primarily be aimed at parents in order to improve vegetable availability at home and to encourage them to promote vegetable preferences.

Acknowledgement

This study is being carried out with financial support from the Commission of the European Communities, specific RTD programme 'Quality of Life and Management of Living Resources', QLK1-2001-00547 'Promoting and Sustaining Health through Increased Fruit and Vegetable Consumption among European Schoolchildren' (Pro Children). The study does not necessarily reflect the Commission's views and in no way anticipates the Commission's future policy in this area.

References

1 Klepp K-I, Pérez-Rodrigo C, De Bourdeaudhuij I, Due P, Elmadfa I, Haraldsdóttir J, König J, Sjöström M, Thórsdóttir I, de Almeida MDV, Yngve A, Brug J: Promoting fruit and vegetable consumption among European schoolchildren: rationale, conceptualization and design of the Pro Children Project. Ann Nutr Metab 2005;49:212–220.

2 Bartholomew KL, Parcel GS, Kok G, Gottlieb NH: Intervention Mapping: Designing Theory- and Evidence-Based Health Promotion Programs. Mountain View, Mayfield Publishing Company, 2001.

3 Green LW, Kreuter MW: Health Promotion Planning: An Educational and Ecological Approach, ed 3. Mountain View, Mayfield, 1999.

4 Gibson EL, Wardle J, Watts CJ: Fruit and vegetable consumption, nutritional knowledge and beliefs in mothers and children. Appetite 1998;31:205–228.

5 Bere E, Klepp KI: Correlates of fruit and vegetable intake among Norwegian schoolchildren: parental and self-reports. Public Health Nutr 2004;7:991–998.

6 Roos EB, Hirvonen T, Mikkilä V, Karvonen S, Rimpela M: Household educational level as a determinant of consumption of raw vegetables among male and female adolescents. Prev Med 2001;33:282–291.

7 Perez-Rodrigo C, Ribas L, Serra-Majem L, Aranceta J: Food preferences of Spanish children and young people: the enKid study. Eur J Clin Nutr 2003;57:S45–S48.

8 Martens M, van Assema P, Brug J: Why do adolescents eat what they eat? Personal and social environmental predictors of fruit, snack and breakfast consumption among Dutch 12- to 14-year-old students. Public Health Nutr, in press.

9 Osler M, Hansen ET: Dietary knowledge and behaviour among schoolchildren in Copenhagen, Denmark. Scand J Soc Med 1993;21:135–140.

10 Cullen KW, Baranowski T, Rittenberry L, Olvera N: Social-environmental influences on children's diets: results from focus groups with African-, Euro- and Mexican-American children and their parents. Health Educ Res 2000;15:581–590.

11 Baranowski T, Domel S, Gould R, Baranowski J, Leonard S, Treiber F, Mullis R: Increasing fruit and vegetable consumption among 4th and 5th grade students: results from focus groups using reciprocal determinism. J Nutr Educ 1993;25:114–120.

12 Bauer KW, Yang YW, Austin SB: 'How can we stay healthy when you're throwing all of this in front of us?' Findings from focus groups and interviews in middle schools on environmental influences on nutrition and physical activity. Health Educ Behav 2004;31:34–46.

13 Morgan DL, Krueger RA: The Focus Group Kit. Thousand Oaks, Sage, 1998.
14 Vaugh S, Schumm JS, Sinagub J: Focus Group Interviews in Education and Psychology. Thousand Oaks, Sage, 1996.
15 Kidd PS, Parshall MB: Getting the focus and the group: enhancing analytical rigor in focus group research. Qual Health Res 2000;10:293–308.
16 Morrison-Beedy D, Cote-Arsenault D, Feinstein NF: Maximizing results with focus groups: moderator and analysis issues. Appl Nurs Res 2001;14:48–53.
17 Baranowski T, Cullen KW, Baranowski J: Psychosocial correlates of dietary intake: advancing dietary intervention. Annu Rev Nutr 1999; 19:17–40.
18 Brug J, Lechner L, De Vries H: Psychosocial determinants of fruit and vegetable consumption. Appetite 1995;25:85–296.
19 Glanz K, Lewis FM, Rimer BK: Health Behaviour and Health Education: Theory, Research and Practice, ed 3. San Francisco, Jossey-Bass, 2002.
20 Conner M, Norman P: Predicting Health Behaviour. Philadelphia, Open University Press, 1996.
21 Baranowski T, Cullen KW, Nicklas T, Thompson D, Baranowski J: Are current health behavioural change models helpful in guiding prevention of weight gain efforts? Obes Res 2003; 11:23S–43S.
22 Story M, Neumark-Sztainer D, French S: Individual and environmental influences on adolescent eating behaviours. J Am Diet Assoc 2002;102:S40–S51.
23 Kratt P, Reynolds K, Shewchuk R: The role of availability as a moderator of family fruit and vegetable consumption. Health Educ Behav 2000;27:471–482.
24 Baranowski T, Lin LS, Wetter DW, Resnicow K, Hearn MD: Theory as mediating variables: why aren't community interventions working as desired? Ann Epidemiol 1997;7:S89–S95.
25 Quality Imaging Products: QSR NVivo. Version 1.3, Australia, 1999–2002.
26 De Bourdeaudhuij I: Family Variables and Health Behaviours in Adolescents, with Focus on Nutrition. Ghent, Ghent University, 1997.
27 Vereecken C, Maes L: Eating habits, dental care and dieting; in Currie C, Hurrelman K, Settertobulte R, Smith R, Todd J (eds): Health and Health Behaviour among Young People. Copenhagen, World Health Organization, 2000.
28 Kremers SP, Brug J, de Vries H, Engels RC: Parenting style and adolescent fruit consumption. Appetite 2003;41:43–50.
29 Bogers R, Brug J, van Assema P, Dagnelie PC: Explaining fruit and vegetable consumption: the theory of planned behaviour and misconception of personal intake levels. Appetite 2004;42:157–166.
30 Vereecken CA, Bobelijn K, Maes L: School food policy at primary and secondary schools in Belgium-Flanders: does it influence young people's food habits? Eur J Clin Nutr 2005;59: 217–7.
31 Pijpers FIM, Van Rijckevorsel JLA, Vogels AGC: Verschillen basisscholen in gezondheidsbeleid? Tijdschr Soc Gezondheidsz 1999; 77:261–266.
32 Shepherd J, Harden A, Rees R, Brunton G, Garcia J, Oliver S, Oakley A: Young people and healthy eating: a systematic review of research on barriers and facilitators. London, EPPI-Centre, University of London, 2001, pp 1–194.
33 Anonymous: Zo eet Nederland. Den Haag, Voedingscentrum, 1998.
34 De Bourdeaudhuij I, Klepp K-I, Due P, Perez Rodrigo C, De Almeida MDV, Wind M, Krølner R, Sandvik C, Brug J: Reliability and validity of a questionnaire to measure personal, social and environmental correlates of fruit and vegetable intake in 10- to 11-year-old children in five European countries. Public Health Nutr 2005;8:129–200.
35 Booth SL, Sallis JF, Ritenbaugh C, Hill JO, Birch LL, Frank LD, Glanz K, Himmelgreen DA, Mudd M, Popkin BM, et al: Environmental and societal factors affect food choice and physical activity: rationale, influences, and leverage points. Nutr Rev 2001;59:S21–S39.
36 French SA, Stables G: Environmental interventions to promote vegetable and fruit consumption among youth in school settings. Prev Med 2003;37:593–610.
37 Cullen KW, Baranowski T, Owens E, Marsh T, Rittenberry L, de Moor C: Availability, accessibility, and preferences for fruit, 100% fruit juice, and vegetables influence children's dietary behaviour. Health Educ Behav 2003;30: 615–626.

Annals of
Nutrition&
Metabolism

Ann Nutr Metab 2005;49:236–245
DOI: 10.1159/000087247

Published online: July 28, 2005

Fruit and Vegetable Intake in a Sample of 11-Year-Old Children in 9 European Countries: The Pro Children Cross-Sectional Survey

Agneta Yngve[a] Alexandra Wolf[b] Eric Poortvliet[a] Ibrahim Elmadfa[b] Johannes Brug[c] Bettina Ehrenblad[a] Bela Franchini[d] Jóhanna Haraldsdóttir[e] Rikke Krølner[f] Lea Maes[g] Carmen Pérez-Rodrigo[h] Michael Sjöström[a] Inga Thórsdóttir[i,j] Knut-Inge Klepp[k]

[a]Department of Biosciences, Unit for Preventive Nutrition, Karolinska Institutet, Stockholm, Sweden; [b]Institute for Nutritional Sciences, University of Vienna, Vienna, Austria; [c]Department of Public Health, Erasmus University Medical Center Rotterdam, Rotterdam, The Netherlands; [d]Faculty of Nutrition and Food Sciences, University of Porto, Porto, Portugal; [e]Research Department of Human Nutrition, Royal Veterinary and Agricultural University, and [f]Department of Social Medicine, Institute of Public Health, Faculty of Health Sciences, University of Copenhagen, Copenhagen, Denmark; [g]Department of Public Health, Ghent University, Ghent, Belgium; [h]Community Nutrition Unit, Bilbao, Spain; [i]Unit for Nutrition Research, Landspitali University Hospital, and [j]Department of Food Science, University of Iceland, Reykjavik, Iceland; [k]Department of Nutrition, Faculty of Medicine, University of Oslo, Oslo, Norway

Key Words

European schoolchildren · Fruit intake · Vegetable intake · 24-Hour recall · Food frequency · Pro Children study

Abstract

Background/Aims: An adequate fruit and vegetable intake provides essential nutrients and nutritive compounds and is considered an important part of a healthy lifestyle. No simple instrument has been available for the assessment of fruit and vegetable intake as well as its determinants in school-aged children applicable in different European countries. Within the Pro Children Project, such an instrument has been developed. This paper describes the cross-sectional survey in 11-year-olds in 9 countries. ***Methods:*** The cross-sectional survey used nationally, and in 2 countries regionally, representative samples of schools and classes. The questionnaires, including a precoded 24-hour recall component and a food frequency part, were completed in the classroom. Data were treated using common syntax files for portion sizes and for merging of vegetable types into four subgroups. ***Results:*** The results show that the fruit and vegetable intake in amounts and choice were highly diverse in the 9 participating countries. Vegetable intake was in general lower than fruit intake, boys consumed less fruit and vegetables than girls did. The highest total intake according to the 24-hour recall was found in Austria and Portugal, the lowest in Spain and Iceland. ***Conclusion:*** The fruit and vegetable intake in 11-year-old children was in all countries far from reaching population goals and food-based dietary guidelines on national and international levels.

Introduction

For promotion of eating habits which are in line with recent food-based dietary guidelines [1–4], it is important to have valid and reliable, simple assessment tools avail-

KARGER

Fax +41 61 306 12 34
E-Mail karger@karger.ch
www.karger.com

© 2005 S. Karger AG, Basel
0250–6807/05/0494–0236$22.00/0

Accessible online at:
www.karger.com/anm

Agneta Yngve
Unit for Preventive Nutrition, Department of Biosciences, Novum
SE–141 57 Huddinge (Sweden)
Tel. +46 8 608 9209, +46 70 550 6557 (mobile), Fax +46 8 608 3350
E-Mail agneta.yngve@prevnut.ki.se

Table 1. WHO population goal[1] and national food-based dietary guidelines for fruit and vegetable intake

Country	Recommendation			Comments
	fruit	vegetables	total	
WHO Europe			≥400g	tubers excluded; all age groups included
Austria	250 g	250 g	5 times/day	potatoes excluded; for 10- to 12-year-olds
Belgium	1–3 portions	300 g		juice and potatoes excluded; from 6 years and onwards
Denmark	3 portions	3 portions	600 g	potatoes excluded, juice included as maximum one portion; for children from 10 years and above and adults; portions used for evaluation of intake
Iceland	>200 g	>200 g	500 g	potatoes excluded, fruit juice included in total; all age groups
Netherlands	2 pieces of fruit	150 g		potatoes excluded; one piece of fruit can be taken as juice; a piece equals approx. 125 g of fruit, or one apple
Norway	2 portions	3 portions	750 g	potatoes and fruit juice included; for adults; same number of portions for children although smaller
Portugal	3–5 portions	3–5 portions		potatoes excluded; portions used for evaluation of energy/calories intake: 3–5 portions for 2,200 kcal – general population; 5 for >3,000 kcal
Spain	3 portions	2 portions	≥400 g	potatoes and fruit juice excluded; same number of portions for children although smaller; portions used for evaluation of intake
Sweden			≥400–500 g	potatoes excluded, fruit juice counted as maximum 100 g; 400 g for children up to 10; 500 for all >10 years of age

[1] Population intake goals represent the population average intake that is judged to be consistent with the maintenance of health in a population.

able. No such assessment tool exists in Europe for use in cross-national comparisons. During the last decades, an increasing amount of attention has been paid to the importance of a high fruit and vegetable intake as an essential part of a healthy lifestyle [1, 2]. The importance of fruit and vegetables for providing essential nutrients such as folate, vitamin C and β-carotene has been emphasized by several reports [1–5], as well as for providing antioxidants of nonvitamin nature and so-called phytoestrogens [1–5]. A number of international recommendations [1, 3, 4] and population targets [2] have been published regarding the desirable level of consumption of fruit and vegetables for adults. A summary of the range reported in the national food-based dietary guidelines for fruit and vegetable intake in the European region is 'more than 400–600 g per day' [6], where the range stands for the variability between countries. The WHO population goal [3] for fruit and vegetable intake is 400 g per day. National food-based dietary guidelines for adults can be found in all investigated countries [3, 7–15], specific guidelines for children exist in some of the investigated countries [3, 7, 10–13, 15–17] (table 1). The guidelines in some cases include suggestions for how they can be used to evaluate intakes.

Fruit and vegetable intake of children has not been extensively monitored on the European level, but has been studied in some national [18–20] surveys. There have been attempts to quantify the intake of individual members of the household from household budget surveys [21], thereby providing possibilities for identifying the fruit and vegetable intake of children. The Health Behaviour in School-Aged Children Study [22] has collected data on fruit and vegetable intake through a simple food frequency questionnaire since 1985. A common protocol for a slightly more sophisticated method of investigating the fruit and vegetable intake in schoolchildren has been missing in the European context.

The Pro Children Project

The Pro Children cross-sectional survey was designed to provide information on actual levels of fruit and veg-

Table 2. Sample selection, response rates, dropout and data cleaning description by country

Country	Partici-pants	Response rate		Dropout rate		Data entry		Data included in the analyses		
		n	% of part	n	% of part	n	% of part	n	% of part	% of data entry
Norway	1,347	1,205	89.5	9	0.7	1,196	88.8	1,157	85.9	96.7
Spain	1,410	1,335	94.7	22	1.6	1,313	93.1	1,289	91.4	98.2
Iceland	1,392	1,235	88.7	39	2.8	1,196	85.9	1,176	84.5	98.3
Denmark	2,111	1,942	92.0	23	1.1	1,919	90.9	1,859	88.1	96.9
Portugal	2,535	2,494	98.4	360	14.2	2,134	84.2	2,118	83.6	99.3
Austria	1,857	1,769	95.3	77	4.1	1,692	91.1	1,656	89.1	97.9
Netherlands	1,396	1,113	79.7	8	0.6	1,105	79.2	1,096	78.5	99.2
Sweden	1,752	1,476	84.2	69	3.9	1,407	80.3	1,364	77.9	96.9
Belgium	1,604	1,355	84.5	12	0.7	1,343	83.7	1,322	82.4	98.4
Total	15,404	13,924	90.4	619	4.0	13,305	86.4	13,037	84.6	98.0

part = Participants.

etable intake among European schoolchildren and their parents as well as the determinants of such consumption patterns. The Pro Children cross-sectional survey constitutes the first ever cross-national comparison of fruit and vegetable intake performed in children, while including determinants (cultural, socioeconomic, and sociocognitive factors). The large variation seen in eating habits across Europe, including practices related to the fruit and vegetable intake, made it particularly important to conduct such a study.

The main objective of the present paper was to describe the results of the Pro Children cross-sectional survey with regard to the total fruit and vegetable intake and frequency of consumption in children in all the participating countries, compared to relevant dietary guidelines.

Method

The cross-sectional survey of the schoolchildren and their parents was conducted in all 9 countries during October to December 2003. Schools constituted the sampling unit, and from each country samples of at least 20 schools and a minimum of 1,300 eligible children were included. The student sample size was seen as sufficient to allow for the planned within-country comparisons (gender, socioeconomic status and urban-rural differences) and take the school component of the variance into account. The target group was children born in 1992. Nationally statistically representative samples of schools were drawn in each country with the exception of Austria and Belgium. For Austria, the sample is statistically representative of the eastern region (population of approximately 4 million; 42% of total population). For Belgium, the sample is statistically representative of Flanders (the Dutch-speaking north-western half of the country, population of approximately 6 million, 58% of total population). The response rates, dropouts and incomplete questionnaires rejected during data cleaning are described in table 2, while the age and gender distribution of the final sample is described in table 3. Only 1.7% of the 24-hour recall (0.6 girls/1.1 boys) and 1.9% of the food frequency (0.9 girls/1.0 boys) questionnaires were excluded from the analysis due to incomplete answers in the dietary intake part of the questionnaire.

The Instrument

A comprehensive survey instrument assessing fruit and vegetable intake and psychosocial factors associated with these consumption patterns was developed for both pupils and their parents. The instruments were originally developed in English prior to translation into the relevant languages within each participating country. These national versions were then back-translated into English by language-proficient individuals not involved in the development of the instruments.

The dietary questionnaire comprises two sections: a precoded 24-hour recall component asking in detail about yesterday's fruit and vegetable intake, and a food frequency part with 5 questions on usual fruit and vegetable intake. The 24-hour recall component was used for measuring group mean intake and for specifying the type of fruits and vegetables eaten, whereas the food frequency part was used for ranking subjects according to their usual intake. The instrument is further described by Haraldsdottir et al. [23]. Multiple pilot tests, including reliability and validity testing, were conducted in a number of countries before the final instrument was decided upon [23]. Based on formal testing of the child instruments in Belgium, Denmark, Iceland, Norway and Portugal, it was concluded that the questionnaire instrument was valid and reliable in giving national group means of fruit and vegetable intake among 11-year-old children as well as ranking them by intake.

The Procedure

The headmasters of the schools were approached about their willingness to participate, and the class teachers were asked to col-

Table 3. Age and gender distribution of the final sample by country and total

Country	Total			Girls			Boys			
	n	age	SD	n	age	SD	n	age	SD	% boys
Austria	1,656	11.0	0.59	871	11.0	0.59	785	11.1	0.60	47.4
Belgium	1,322	11.5	0.46	606	11.5	0.46	716	11.5	0.46	54.2
Denmark	1,859	11.4	0.38	918	11.3	0.35	941	11.4	0.39	50.6
Iceland	1,176	11.3	0.33	562	11.3	0.34	614	11.3	0.31	52.2
Netherlands	1,096	11.7	0.46	590	11.7	0.44	506	11.8	0.48	46.2
Norway	1,157	11.3	0.32	569	11.3	0.32	588	11.3	0.31	50.8
Portugal	2,118	11.5	0.45	1,115	11.5	0.43	1,003	11.5	0.47	0.47
Spain	1,289	11.4	0.44	599	11.4	0.41	690	11.4	0.46	53.5
Sweden	1,364	11.4	0.47	687	11.4	0.47	677	11.4	0.46	49.6
Total	13,037	11.4	0.48	6,517	11.3	0.47	6,520	11.4	0.48	50.0

lect the data using standardized instructions. The data for the children's intake were collected directly in the classroom using the validated instrument. Data were entered at the national centers, according to a standardized protocol, prior to submission to the joint Data Management Centre at the University of Vienna, where data processing and quality control has taken place.

Data Treatment

The results from the 24-hour recalls regarding vegetables were merged into four subgroups, i.e. salad, raw vegetables, cooked vegetables and soup vegetables, in order to provide useful information for the design of interventions. The results from the food frequency questionnaire were converted to 'once a day or more' regarding frequency of total fruit and vegetable intake. Portion sizes were corrected for differences in standard servings between countries, in particular for cucumber and carrots (due to different slicing habits for pieces or slices). A maximum number of portions consumed per meal was determined for each fruit and vegetable item and intakes were adjusted using a standardized script. The results were tested for age-related differences. As no such differences could be identified, the results are presented only according to gender and country.

Research Clearance

The cross-sectional survey involves children (9–13 years of age) and their parents (healthy volunteers). Self-administered questionnaires are the only research instruments used. Parental written consent was obtained prior to including the children in the cross-sectional survey. Furthermore, research clearance was obtained from research ethics committees in all countries where this was regulated for this kind of noninvasive study.

Data Analysis

Data analysis was conducted using the program software Statistical Package for Social Sciences 12.0 (SPSS). For age and gender differences, statistical significance was established as $p < 0.05$. Nonparametric Mann-Whitney U tests corrected with Shaffer were used, due to the absence of normal distribution of consumption data even after logarithmic transformation.

Results

24-Hour Recall

Fruit, fruit juice, vegetable, as well as added fruit and vegetable intake are presented in table 4a–d. Girls had a significantly higher fruit, vegetable and total fruit and vegetable intake than boys ($p < 0.000$) and a slightly higher fruit juice intake, though not significant ($p = 0.098$). A large variation in consumption was found between the countries. The highest overall fruit intakes were found in Austria, Denmark and Portugal (171, 157 and 153 g). Fruit intakes were lowest in Iceland and Spain (90 and 118 g). Children in Portugal, Sweden and Belgium showed the highest overall vegetable intakes in this study (mean 111, 109 and 105 g). The countries with the lowest vegetable intakes were Iceland and Spain (mean 54 and 58 g). The highest overall fruit and vegetable intakes were found in Austria and Portugal (265 and 264 g), while the lowest intakes were found in Iceland and Spain (143 and 176 g). The highest juice intakes were found in Austria and the Netherlands (360 and 267 g), the lowest in Portugal and Denmark (142 and 143 g).

Figure 1 presents the average fruit intake in grams per day per country. Figure 2 shows vegetable intake in grams/day per country indicating the type of vegetables eaten. Raw vegetables were consumed much more in the northern countries. In Portugal and Spain, the main intake of vegetables came from vegetable soup.

Food Frequency Questionnaire

The food frequency data are presented in figures 3 and 4. The percentage of children choosing the alternatives

Table 4. The 24-hour recall (P = percentile)

a Fruit intake (g)

Country	Total						Girls		Boys	
	mean	95% CI	median	P25	P75	P90	mean	median	mean	median
Austria	171	163–179	150	0	250	400	171	125	171	150
Belgium	137	130–145	100	0	200	300	142	100	133	100
Denmark	157	150–164	100	0	200	400	168	150	146	100
Iceland	90	83–96	50	0	100	250	87	50	93	50
Netherlands	134	126–142	100	0	200	300	142	100	125	100
Norway	149	140–158	100	0	200	375	157	100	141	100
Portugal	153	147–158	150	50	200	300	152	150	153	125
Spain	118	111–125	100	0	200	300	117	100	118	100
Sweden	129	122–136	100	0	200	300	134	100	125	100
Total	141	138–143	100	0	200	300	144	100	137	100

b Juice intake (g)

Country	mean	95% CI	median	P25	P75	P90	Girls mean	Girls median	Boys mean	Boys median
Austria	360	343–378	300	0	600	800	348	300	375	400
Belgium	225	210–240	200	0	400	600	215	200	234	200
Denmark	143	133–154	0	0	200	400	144	0	142	0
Iceland	211	197–225	200	0	400	600	200	200	221	200
Netherlands	267	250–284	200	0	400	600	287	200	244	200
Norway	195	179–211	0	0	400	600	207	100	184	0
Portugal	142	133–150	0	0	200	400	135	0	150	0
Spain	213	202–225	200	0	400	500	212	200	214	200
Sweden	197	182–212	0	0	400	600	186	0	209	0
Total	213	208–217	200	0	400	600	209	200	215	200

c Vegetable intake (g)

Country	mean	95% CI	median	P25	P75	P90	Girls mean	Girls median	Boys mean	Boys median
Austria	94	89–99	60	0	140	240	99	60	88	60
Belgium	105	100–110	80	30	150	235	101	80	108	80
Denmark	84	79–89	40	0	125	231	92	60	76	40
Iceland	54	49–59	10	0	70	165	57	30	50	0
Netherlands	70	65–75	60	0	100	160	73	60	67	60
Norway	67	62–73	30	0	105	195	75	40	60	10
Portugal	111	107–115	80	30	160	250	112	90	110	80
Spain	58	54–62	40	0	80	160	56	40	60	40
Sweden	109	103–115	75	20	155	265	118	80	100	65
Total	86	85–88	60	0	130	220	90	60	83	60

d Fruit plus vegetable intake (g)

Country	mean	95% CI	median	P25	P75	P90	Girls mean	Girls median	Boys mean	Boys median
Austria	265	254–275	210	100	390	590	269	220	259	200
Belgium	242	232–252	200	100	340	500	243	210	242	200
Denmark	241	231–250	200	80	350	535	260	215	222	180
Iceland	143	134–153	100	0	200	350	144	100	143	100
Netherlands	204	194–214	165	100	284	430	214	180	193	160
Norway	216	204–228	160	60	315	505	232	200	201	143
Portugal	264	256–271	240	130	361	500	264	240	263	240
Spain	176	168–185	145	50	250	390	174	150	179	140
Sweden	238	228–249	200	93	340	500	251	225	225	190
Total	227	224–230	190	80	330	500	235	200	219	180

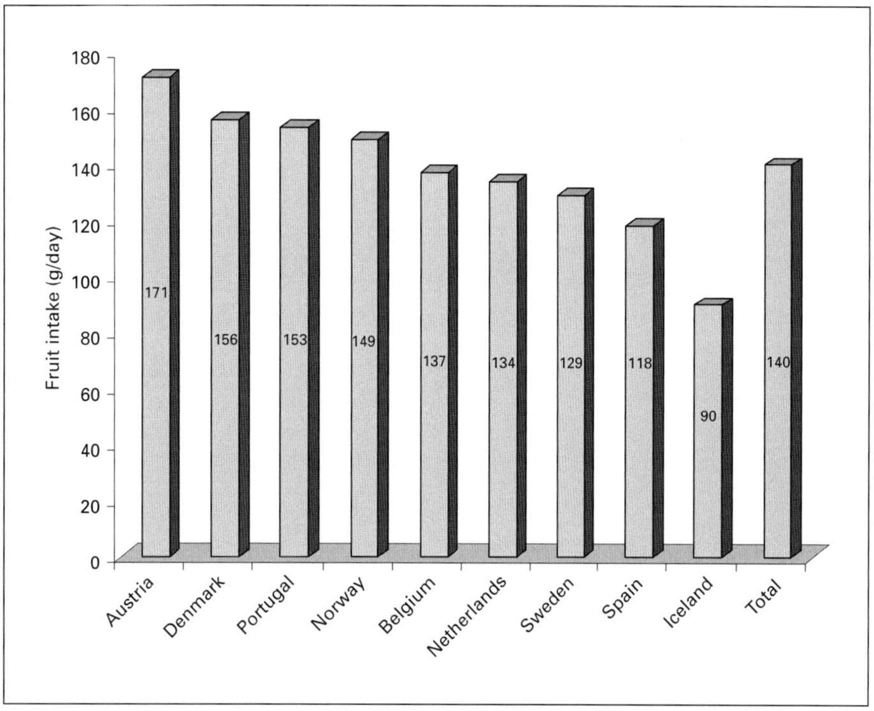

Fig. 1. Mean consumption of fruit (g/day).

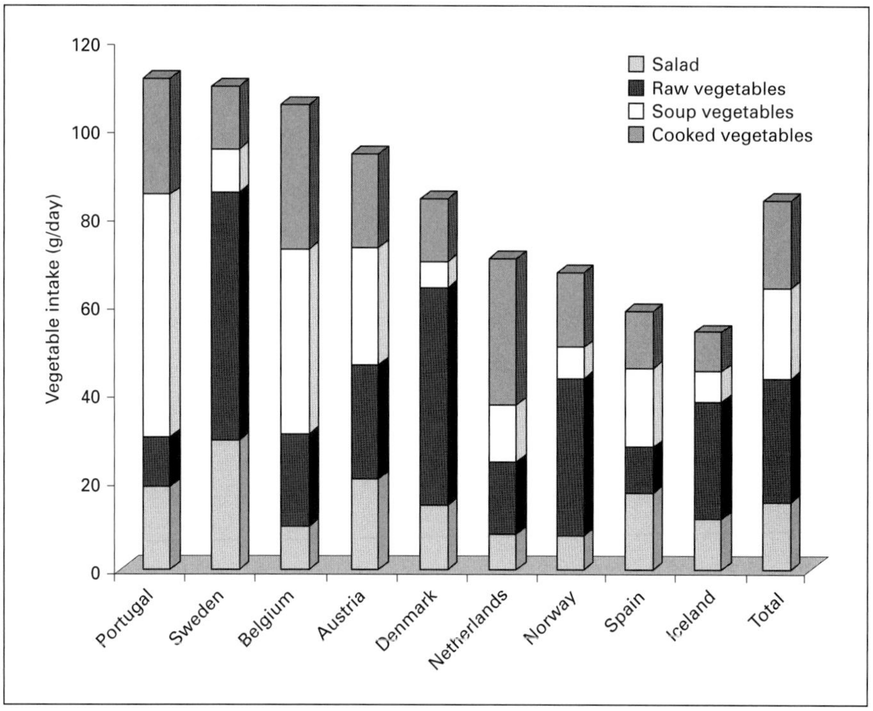

Fig. 2. Mean consumption of vegetables, shown as subgroups and total (g/day).

once every day, twice every day, more than twice every day for both fruit and vegetable is shown. Less than half of all the investigated children indicated that they eat fruit (48%) or vegetable (45%) every day.

Discussion

Among the 9 European countries participating in this cross-sectional survey, a diverse and complicated picture of fruit and vegetable intake emerged. Children in all

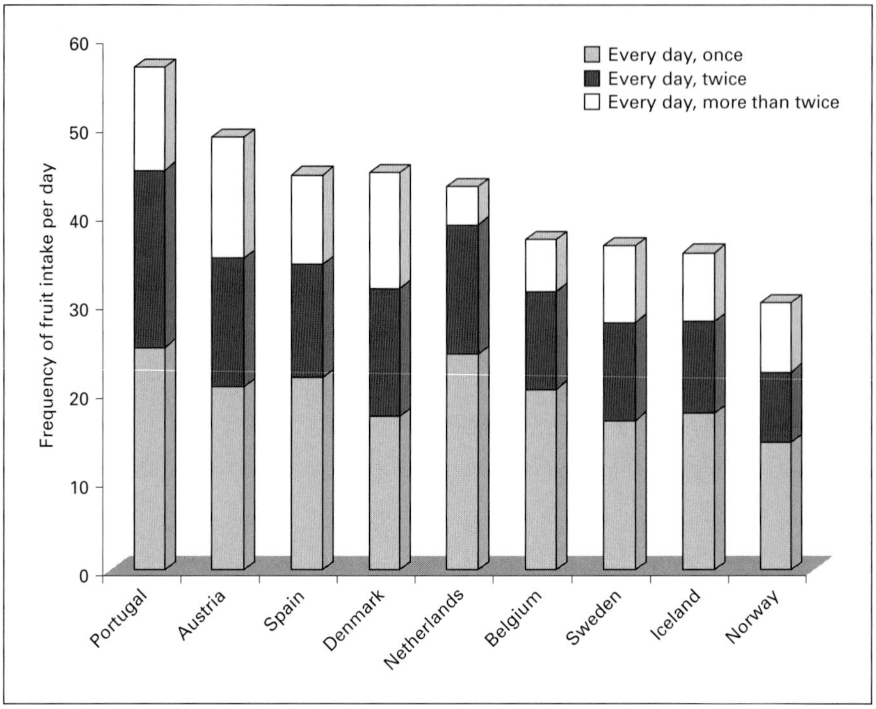

Fig. 3. Frequency of intake of fruit, ≥1 time per day.

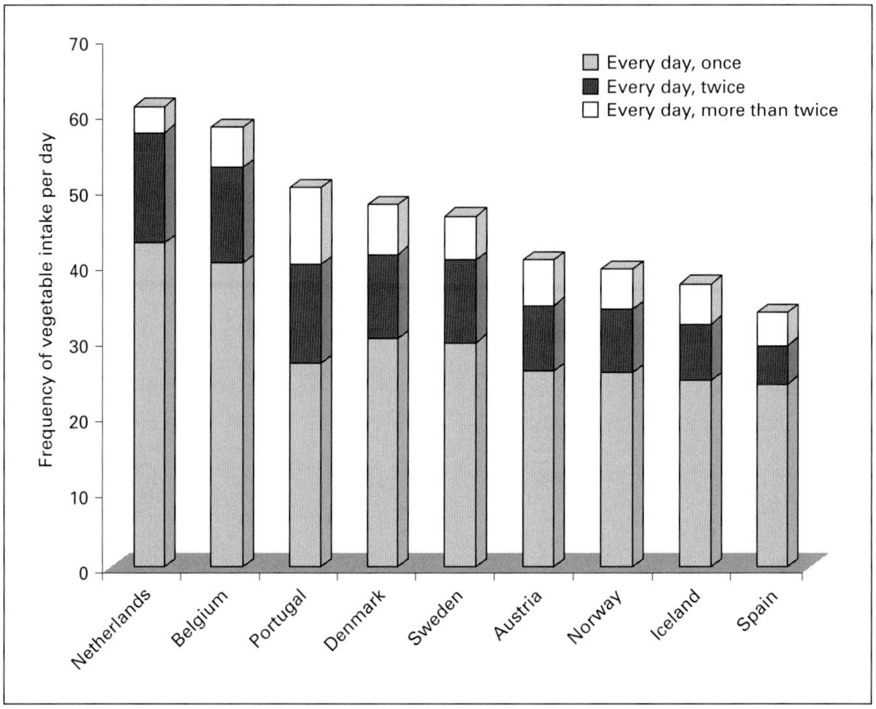

Fig. 4. Frequency of intake of vegetables, ≥1 time per day.

countries showed relatively low intakes of both fruit and vegetables with consistently lower intakes of vegetables. Boys had in general a lower fruit and vegetable intake than girls. There was no clear north-south gradient, except for the type of vegetables eaten (raw vegetables, cooked vegetables and vegetable soup). The higher intake of raw vegetables in the northern countries might reflect different preferences, but could also have been due to culturally dependent factors related to food preparation and availability.

The response rates were overall unusually high, probably due to the use of schools and classes as sampling units. Due to the school-based survey, respondent bias (overrepresentation of healthy, well-educated subjects) was probably lower than in other types of studies. Because of the statistically representative samples in all countries except for Belgium and Austria, the results should be representative for the countries, and for Belgium and Austria for the chosen regions. Comparisons between the countries could however present some problems, due to differences in food culture and perception of portion sizes.

The main limitation of the 24-hour recall in this precoded instrument was that intakes were recorded for one weekday only and therefore did not reflect usual intake. The food frequency questionnaire should to some extent have corrected for this and in comparison, the ranking of countries based on actual intake (24-hour recall) fits rather nicely with the ranking of usual intake (food frequency questionnaire). In Spain, we could, however, see that the ranking for usual intake seemed higher than the actual intake for fruit, and in the Netherlands the ranking for usual intake was higher for vegetables than the one for actual intake. Group averages of weekday intakes were considered relatively reliable due to the narrow age range and such large samples in each country.

Another problem with the instruments was the portion size estimation for carrots and cucumber that was performed by the Pro Children consortium, where the ways of serving these vegetables turned out to be diverse between countries (e.g. sticks of different sizes, thick or thin slices). Also, as was shown in focus groups [24], children in Belgium had problems distinguishing fruit juice from lemonades and other fruit-based drinks, which is why the data on fruit juice should be interpreted with caution.

Fruit juice intake seemed high in some countries, and may have contributed substantially to the intake of vitamin C and folate. Another problem with the survey results was the fact that different vegetables have very different contents of active compounds of nutrients and other potentially nutritionally important components.

In adding up intakes of different kinds of fruits and vegetables to total intake levels, we therefore neglected possibly relevant differences within the fruit and vegetable food groups. We did not include potatoes in the analysis, which might provide substantial amounts of vitamin C in countries where potato consumption is high. Another problem was the season when the data were collected. October and November are in many countries, except for Spain, the period when nationally or locally grown fruit, berries and vegetables are available in vast amounts. This could mean that data for fruit and vegetable intake collected at other times of the year could be even lower, or in the case of Spain that fruit and vegetable intake would be higher if collected at another time of the year.

Generally, the results of the present study were in line with the results from earlier studies on fruit and vegetable intake in the participating countries [9, 19, 25–30] when taking the differences in methodology and year of survey into account. The results of the present study for both fruit and vegetable intake frequency also show roughly the same ranking of countries as the Health Behaviour in School-Aged Children Study [22]. However, data on availability of fruits and vegetables [31, 32] show a north-south gradient, where the southernmost countries had the highest availability; a finding that was not reflected in the present results.

The WHO population goal [3] for consumption of fruit and vegetables (table 1) is 400 g per day. It does not specify whether fruit juice should be included. The WHO population goal represents the population average that is judged to be consistent with the maintenance of health. No clear guidelines on how to interpret the population goal for intake evaluation purposes could be identified. Our analyses indicate that average intakes of children in almost all countries exceeded the population goal of 400 g when our data on fruit juice were included. However, we showed earlier [24] that children of this age had problems distinguishing fruit juice from other fruit drinks or lemonades. After exclusion of juice intake, the results showed that mean intakes of fruit and vegetables in all countries were lower than the WHO population goal. Children in Austria and Portugal, with the highest intakes of fruit and vegetables, both reached a mean intake of about 264 g per day.

No guidelines for how to interpret population goals for this specific age group were identified either. Possibly, children of this age group should end up somewhere in the lower end of the range compared with the range of intake for the whole population. Due to this problem, it was even more difficult to judge to which extent the population of children in this study achieved the WHO population goal.

An attempt was made to use a British example [33] of identifying compliers and noncompliers of the WHO population goal of 400 g. This was done by ranking the sum of vegetable and fruit intake and selecting a cutoff point when the group mean reached 400 g. The cutoff applied in the total group was 210 g, depending on the distribution of intake. In the total sample, the resulting per-

Table 5. Percentage of 11-year-old children with fruit plus vegetable intake ≥ 400 g, by gender and country

Country	Total		Girls		Boys	
	n	%	n	%	n	%
Austria	400	24.1	212	24.3	188	23.9
Belgium	253	19.1	108	17.8	145	20.3
Denmark	394	21.2	218	23.7	176	18.7
Iceland	92	7.8	36	6.4	56	9.1
Netherlands	130	11.9	77	13.1	53	10.5
Norway	202	17.5	109	19.2	93	15.8
Portugal	453	21.4	227	20.4	226	22.5
Spain	125	9.7	45	7.5	80	11.6
Sweden	250	18.3	136	19.7	114	16.8
Total	2,299	17.6	1,168	17.9	1,131	17.3

centage of compliers (which should be 100% if the population goal was achieved) was 44.5%. Among the compliers, there were more girls than boys in all countries except for Spain. If, on the other hand, the 400 g population goal is used as a cutoff for fruit and vegetable intake, we can see that the percentage of 11-year-olds in the 9 countries that eat 400 g of fruits and vegetables per day varies between 6.4 and 24.3%, depending on gender and country (table 5).

National recommendations were in most cases higher than the WHO population goal (table 1). In some countries, fruit juice without limitation was included in the recommendation, while other countries allowed the inclusion of one portion of fruit juice per day, interpreted as 100 g. Yet other countries did not include fruit juice at all. In all countries, except for Norway, potatoes were excluded from the recommendations. Some countries used the same recommendations for adults and children. The recommendations sometimes included guidelines for interpretation of survey results; Spain, Denmark and Portugal specified that portions were supposed to be used for evaluation of intake. When taking all these factors into account, the average intake in all countries failed to reach the own nationally recommended levels in this study.

For those countries which used portions for evaluating intake, 6.0 and 5.8% of girls and boys in Denmark, 19.5 and 13.3% in Norway, 23.2 and 22.2% in Portugal and 0.8 and 1.2% in Spain reached the recommended number of portions for fruit and vegetables. Comparison of the Norwegian data with national recommendations was however difficult as potato intake was not measured in this study.

The Dutch and Belgian recommendations are expressed both in grams (for vegetables) and portions (for fruit). For the Netherlands 7.8 and 5.7%, and for Belgium 14.0 and 13.3% of girls and boys, respectively, reached both recommendations for fruit and vegetables.

For Austria 6.4 and 7.6%, for Iceland 3.4 and 4.6% and for Sweden 15.7 and 13.3% of girls and boys reached the recommended intakes, which ranged from 400 to 600 g. According to the National Food Administration in Sweden, the recommendation for fruit and vegetables for Sweden (1/2 kg) should be seen as a population goal, which means that half of the whole population should reach the recommendation.

In the above calculations, fruit juice was not counted at all. This could mean that the results were too pessimistic in many cases, since fruit juice could have contributed to a higher intake of for example folate and vitamin C than indicated by the data on fruit and vegetables.

Conclusions

The average fruit and vegetable intake did not reach WHO population goals or national recommendations in any country when fruit juice was excluded. The fruit and vegetable intake was highly variable across Europe, for total amounts and types of vegetables eaten. Vegetable intake was clearly lower than fruit intake. A large proportion of the investigated group stated a frequency of intake which was less than once a day of fruit and vegetables, respectively.

The future analysis of determinants for fruit and vegetable intake in the Pro Children cross-sectional survey will be of great importance for identifying ways to correct the inadequate intakes that were identified in this analysis.

We can also conclude that there were difficulties in the interpretation of the WHO population goal, since no clear guidelines seemed to exist regarding (1) the inclusion or exclusion of fruit juice and (2) interpretation within selected age groups. Moreover, national recommendations are highly variable and sometimes difficult to interpret.

Acknowledgements

This study is being carried out with financial support from the Commission of the European Communities, specific RTD program 'Quality of Life and Management of Living Resources', QLK1-

2001-00547 'Promoting and Sustaining Health through Increased Vegetable and Fruit Consumption among European Schoolchildren' (Pro Children). The study does not necessarily reflect the Commission's views and in no way anticipates its future policy in this area. Special thanks to all the teachers, headmasters and above all, the children who took the time to participate in this survey, to the staff and students from all 9 participating countries who have collected and entered the data, to Professor Emeritus Leif Hambraeus who advised on the interpretation of results and finally to Emma Patterson who checked the English and gave good advice.

References

1 World Health Organization: Global Strategy on Diet, Physical Activity and Health. Geneva, World Health Organization, 2004.
2 Nutrition and diet for healthy lifestyles in Europe: science and policy implications. Proceedings of the European Conference, May 18–20, 2000, Crete, Greece. Public Health Nutr 2001; 4:337–434.
3 Diet, nutrition and the prevention of chronic diseases. World Health Organ Tech Rep Ser 2003;916:i–viii,1–149,backcover.
4 American Institute for Cancer Research: Food, Nutrition and the Prevention of Cancer: A Global Perspective. Washington, American Institute for Cancer Research, 1997.
5 Klerk M, Jansen CJF, van't Veer P, Kok FJ: Fruits and Vegetables in Chronic Disease Prevention. Wageningen, Division of Human Nutrition and Epidemiology, Wageningen Agricultural University, 1995.
6 World Health Organization: Food-Based Dietary Guidelines in WHO European Member States. Copenhagen, WHO Regional Office for Europe, 2002.
7 Trolle E, Fagt S, Ovesen L: Fruit and vegetables, recommendations for intake; in: Danish Veterinary and Food Administration C. Copenhagen, Quickly Tryk A/S, 1998.
8 Deutsche Gesellschaft für Ernährung, Österreichische Gesellschaft für Ernährung, Schweizerische Gesellschaft für Ernährungsforschung, Schweizerische Vereinigung für Ernährung: Referenzwerte für die Nährstoffzufuhr, ed 1, corr reprint 2. Frankfurt, Umschau Braus GmbH, 2001.
9 Steingrimsdottir L, Thorgeirsdottir H, Olafsdottir AS: The Diet of Icelanders. Dietary Survey of the Icelandic Nutrition Council 2002: Main Findings. Reykjavik, Icelandic Nutrition Council, 2003.
10 Blomhoff R, Lande B, Ose T: Recommendations for Increased Intake of Fruit and Vegetables. Oslo, National Nutrition Council, 1996.
11 Zo eet Nederland. Den Haag, Voedingscentrum, 1998.
12 A nova roda dos alimentos. Uma guia para escolha alimentar diaria! Coma bem, viva melhor. Porto, Garra, Faculdade de Ciencias da Nutricao e Alimentacao da Universidade do Porto, Instituto do Consumidor, 2003.
13 Aranceta J, Serra-Majem L: Dietary guidelines for the Spanish population. Public Health Nutr 2001;4:1403–1408.
14 Ett halvt kilo om dagen! Uppsala, Livsmedelsverket, 2003.
15 Institute FHP: The Flemish Food Guide Pyramid. Ghent, Institute FHP, 2004.
16 Kersting M, Alexy U, Rothmann N: Fakten zur Kinderernährung. München, Hans Marseille Verlag , 2003, p 72.
17 Recommendations for Fruit and Vegetable Intake for Children. Uppsala, Statens Livsmedelsverk, 2004.
18 Perez-Rodrigo C, Ribas L, Serra-Majem L, Aranceta J: Food preferences of Spanish children and young people: the enKid study. Eur J Clin Nutr 2003;57(Suppl 1):S45–S48.
19 Andersen LF, Overby N, Lillegaard IT: Intake of fruit and vegetables among Norwegian children and adolescents. Tidsskr Nor Laegeforen 2004;124:1396–1398.
20 Eriksen K, Haraldsdottir J, Pederson R, Flyger HV: Effect of a fruit and vegetable subscription in Danish schools. Public Health Nutr 2003;6: 57–63.
21 Vasdeki VG, Stylianou S, Naska A: Estimation of age- and gender-specific food availability from household budget survey data. Public Health Nutr 2001;4:1149–1151.
22 Young People's Health in Context: International report from the HBSC 2001/02; in Currie C (ed): Health Policy Series: Health Policy for Children and Adolescents Issue 4. Copenhagen, WHO Regional Office for Europe, 2004.
23 Haraldsdóttir J, Thórsdóttir I, de Almeida MDV, Maes L, de Rodrigues C, Elmadfa I, Andersen LF: Validity and reproducibility of a precoded questionnaire to assess fruit and vegetable intake in European 11- to 12-year-old schoolchildren. Ann Nutr Metab 2005;49: 221–227.
24 Wind M, Bobelijn K, De Bourdeaudhuij I, Klepp K-I, Brug J: A qualitative exploration of determinants of fruit and vegetable intake among 10- and 11-year-old schoolchildren in the Low Countries. Ann Nutr Metab 2005;49:228–235.
25 Serra-Majem L, Ribas-Barba L, Pérez-Rodrigo C, Roman-Vinas B, Aranceta Bartrina J: Hábitos alimentarios y consumo de alimentos en la población infantil y juvenil española (1998–2000): variables socioeconómicas y geográficas. Med Clin (Barc) 2003;121:126–131.
26 Steingrimsdottir L, Thorgeirsdottir H, Aegisdottir S: Hvad bordar islensk aeska? Könnun á mataraedi ungs skolafolks 1992–1993. Rannsoknir Manneldisrads Islands IV. Reykjavik, Iceland, 1994.
27 Fagt S, Matthiessen J, Trolle E, Lyhne N, Christensen T, Hinsch HJ, Biltoft-Jensen A, Möller A, Daae AS: Danskernes kostvaner 2000–2001. Födevare Rapport 2002:10. København, Födevaredirektoratet, 2002.
28 Becker W: Befolkningens kostvanor och näringsintag i Sverige 1989. Uppsala, Statens Livsmedelsverk, 1994.
29 Riksmaten 1997–1998. Kostvanor och näringsintag i Sverige. Metod- och resultatanalys. Uppsala, Livsmedelsverket, 2002.
30 Andersen A, Due P, Poulsen LH, Rasmussen M: Sundhedsvaner; in Due P, Holstein BE (eds): Skoleboernsundersoegelsen 2002. Koebenhavn, Koebenhavns Universitet, Institut for Folkesundhedsvidenskab, 2003.
31 Trichopoulou A, Naska A: European food availability databank based on household budget surveys: the Data Food Networking initiative. Eur J Public Health 2003;13(3 Suppl):24–28.
32 FAO: Food Balance Sheets, FAOSTAT. Rome, FAO, 2002.
33 Hunt C, Nichols RN, Pryer JA: Who complied with national fruit and vegetable population goals? Eur J Public Health 2000;10:178–184.

Annals of
Nutrition& Metabolism

Ann Nutr Metab 2005;49:246–254
DOI: 10.1159/000087248

Published online: July 28, 2005

Fruit and Vegetable Intake of Mothers of 11-Year-Old Children in Nine European Countries: The Pro Children Cross-Sectional Survey

Alexandra Wolf[a] Agneta Yngve[b] Ibrahim Elmadfa[a] Eric Poortvliet[b] Bettina Ehrenblad[b] Carmen Pérez-Rodrigo[c] Inga Thórsdóttir[d,e] Jóhanna Haraldsdóttir[f] Johannes Brug[g] Lea Maes[h] Maria Daniel Vaz de Almeida[i] Rikke Krølner[j] Knut-Inge Klepp[k]

[a]Institute for Nutritional Sciences, University of Vienna, Vienna, Austria; [b]Department of Biosciences, Unit for Preventive Nutrition, Karolinska Institute, Stockholm, Sweden; [c]Community Nutrition Unit, Bilbao, Spain; [d]Unit for Nutrition Research, Landspitali University Hospital, and [e]Department of Food Science, University of Iceland, Reykjavik, Iceland; [f]Research Department of Human Nutrition, Royal Veterinary and Agricultural University, Copenhagen, Denmark; [g]Department of Public Health, Erasmus University Medical Center, Rotterdam, The Netherlands; [h]Department of Public Health, Ghent University, Ghent, Belgium; [i]Faculty of Nutrition and Food Sciences, University of Porto, Porto, Portugal; [j]Department of Social Medicine, Institute of Public Health, Faculty of Health Sciences, University of Copenhagen, Copenhagen, Denmark; [k]Department of Nutrition, Faculty of Medicine, University of Oslo, Oslo, Norway

Key Words

Women · Fruit and vegetable intake · 24-Hour recall · Food frequency · Pro Children study

Abstract

Objective: To describe and compare fruit and vegetable intakes of mothers of 11-year-old children across Europe. ***Methods:*** Cross-sectional surveys were carried out in 9 European countries in October/November 2003. Self-administered questionnaires assessing fruit and vegetable consumption were used for data collection. The current paper presents dietary intake data obtained by a precoded 24-hour recall and a food frequency questionnaire. ***Results:*** The consumption levels of fruit and vegetables (without fruit juice) were in line with World Health Organization recommendations of ≥400 g/day for only 27% of all participating mothers. Based on both instruments, the Pro Children results showed comparatively high average fruit intake levels in Portugal, Denmark and Sweden (211, 203 and 194 g/day) and the lowest intake in Iceland (97 g/day). High vegetable intake levels were found in Portugal and Belgium (169 and 150 g/day), the lowest in Spain (88 g/day). A south-north gradient could not be observed in the Pro Children study. ***Conclusion:*** Fruit and vegetable intakes are low in mothers of 11-year-olds across Europe. Especially vegetable consumption can be regarded as marginal in most of the studied European countries. A high percentage of mothers indicated to eat fruit and vegetables less than once a day. The results have shown that national and international interventions are necessary to promote fruit and especially vegetable consumption in the European population of mothers.

KARGER

Fax +41 61 306 12 34
E-Mail karger@karger.ch
www.karger.com

0250–6807/05/0494–0246$22.00/0

Accessible online at:
www.karger.com/anm

Ibrahim Elmadfa
University of Vienna, Institute for Nutritional Sciences
Althanstrasse 14
AT–1090 Vienna (Austria)
Tel. +43 1 4277 54911, Fax +43 1 4277 9549, E-Mail ibrahim.elmadfa@univie.ac.at

Table 1. WHO population goal[1] and national food-based dietary guidelines for intake of fruit and vegetables

Country	Recommendation			Comments
	fruit	vegetables	total	
WHO Europe			≥400 g	tubers excluded; all age groups
Austria	250–300 g	400 g	5 a day	potatoes excluded, one piece of fruit can be taken as fruit juice; for adults
Belgium	1–3 portions	300 g		juice and potatoes excluded; from 6 years and onwards
Denmark	3 portions	3 portions	600 g	potatoes excluded, juice included as maximum one portion from 10 years and onwards; portions used for evaluation of intake
Iceland	>200 g	>200 g	500 g	potatoes excluded, fruit juice included in total; schoolchildren and onwards
Netherlands	2 pieces	200 g		potatoes excluded, one portion of fruit can be taken as fruit juice; a piece equals approximately 125 g of fruit or one apple; for adults
Norway	2 portions	3 portions	750 g	potatoes and fruit juice included; for adults
Portugal	3–5 portions	3–5 portions		potatoes excluded; portions used for evaluation of intake: 3–5 for 2,200 kcal – general population; 5 for >3,000 kcal
Spain	3 portions	2 portions	≥400 g	potatoes and fruit juice excluded; portions used for evaluation of intake
Sweden	250 g	250 g	½ kg	potatoes excluded, fruit juice counted as maximum 100 g per day

[1] Population intake goals represent the population average intake that is judged to be consistent with the maintenance of health in a population.

Introduction

Epidemiological and clinical studies in the nutrition field have shown the health benefits of adequate fruit and vegetable consumption. Fruit and vegetables are low in energy but relatively rich in vitamins (especially vitamin C and folate), minerals and other bioactive components which are associated with the prevention of chronic disease [1–4].

Recommendations for adequate fruit and vegetable intake levels have been set by most European countries as well as by international health agencies [5–16]. In summary, these food-based dietary guidelines vary in the range of 400–750 g per day considered as an adequate intake amount (table 1).

It is considered of utmost importance to monitor fruit and vegetable intake as one of the main nutrition quality indicators in the European Health Monitoring Program [17]. However, hardly any cross-European data on fruit and vegetable intake are available to date. In many European countries, the availability and supply of fruit and vegetables has been assessed based on food balance sheets or household budget surveys [18–20]. Intake surveys based on computer-assisted interviews [21, 22] or other methods were conducted mostly at the national level in different European countries [23–36]. Some attempts have been made to review data from these national studies to make international comparisons [37, 38], but a simple, self-administered survey instrument for fruit and vegetable intake across Europe is still lacking.

In order to collect important information about actual consumption levels of 11-year-old children and their parents in all participating countries, the Pro Children cross-sectional survey (CSS) was designed. The current paper describes the results of the Pro Children CSS regarding total fruit and vegetable intake of mothers and other female guardians participating in the survey.

Method

The CSS was carried out in 9 European countries (Austria, Belgium, Denmark, Iceland, the Netherlands, Norway, Portugal, Spain and Sweden) in October/November 2003. The target group for the

Table 2. The Pro Children sample by country and total

Country	Partici-pants	Response rate		Dropout rate		Data entry		Female participants[1]		
		n	% of part	n	% of part	n	% of part	n	% of part	% of data entry
Austria	1,857	1,574	84.8	122	6.6	1,452	78.2	1,275	68.7	87.8
Belgium	1,604	1,287	80.2	58	3.6	1,229	76.6	1,070	66.7	87.1
Denmark	2,111	1,478	70.0	42	2.0	1,436	68.0	1,272	60.3	88.6
Iceland	1,392	998	71.7	18	1.3	980	70.4	838	60.2	85.5
Netherlands	1,396	946	67.8	18	1.3	928	66.5	814	58.3	87.7
Norway	1,347	1,009	74.9	0	0.0	1,009	74.9	838	62.2	83.1
Portugal	2,535	2,114	83.4	454	17.9	1,660	65.5	1,376	54.3	82.9
Spain	1,410	1,089	77.2	63	4.5	1,026	72.8	783	55.5	76.3
Sweden	1,752	1,232	70.3	68	3.9	1,164	66.4	975	55.7	83.8
Total	15,404	11,727	76.1	843	5.5	10,884	70.7	9,241	60.0	84.9

Participants = Part.
[1] 13.1% male participants (n = 1,424) and 2.0% (n = 219) missing gender information.

survey were children born in 1992 and their parents. Representative samples of at least 20 schools covering 1,300 eligible children were drawn in each country. For each participating child, one parent was asked to complete a survey questionnaire. These questionnaires were given to the participating children to take home. Parents themselves could decide which parent was to complete the survey. This led to a gender-related selection bias as the questionnaire was primarily filled out by the parent traditionally responsible for the child's care, i.e., the mothers: only 13% of the questionnaires were filled out by male guardians. Therefore, the analyses for the present paper were restricted to the female participants. The response rates for all parents and the number of cases included in the analyses are presented in table 2.

The Instrument

Self-administered questionnaires were used in all countries. The instrument was translated into national languages and tested for reliability and validity in multiple pilot tests prior to final administration [39, 40].

The dietary part of the questionnaire included two sections.

(1) A precoded 24-hour recall asked in detail about fruit and vegetable intake on the previous day. The recall was divided into three time intervals including several eating occasions. Parents were asked if they had had specific fruits or vegetables (juice, fruit, salad, other raw vegetables, cooked vegetables and vegetable soup) during that time interval. The indicated amounts were translated into standardized portion sizes in grams.

(2) A food frequency questionnaire elicited important information about usual fruit and vegetable intake. Eight answer categories (ranging from 'never' to 'more than twice a day') indicated the usual frequency of intake for fresh fruit and fruit juice as well as for raw and cooked vegetables and salads. All frequencies of 'less than once a week' were summarized as 'nonconsumers'.

In the present paper, the 24-hour recall part is used to show group mean intakes in grams per day, whereas the food frequency part is used to rank subjects according to their usual intake.

Data Collection and Analysis

Collection of the children's questionnaires was carried out directly in the classroom by the class teachers. All participating pupils received a closed envelope with an additional questionnaire to take home and be completed by one of their parents. The only identification that was used for the questionnaires was a numeric code to ensure linkage between the parental and the child questionnaire. The completed parent questionnaires were returned by the children to the classroom teachers, who collected all questionnaires and submitted them to the national research center, with the exception of Denmark, where the parents returned the questionnaires directly to the research center [41].

All data collected in the CSS were entered and double-checked in the national centers. All national data sets were pooled in a joint database at the Data Management Center (University of Vienna), where further data processing and quality control were carried out. All data processing (e.g. data entry, cleaning) was done according to a standardized protocol. Research clearance was obtained from research ethics committees in all countries where this is regulated.

Data analysis was conducted using the program software Statistical Package for Social Sciences 12.0 (SPSS). Descriptive statistics were used to study the level of fruit and vegetable intake. Only 1.1% (n = 101) of the 24-hour recalls and 0.8% (n = 74) of the food frequency questionnaires were excluded due to incompleteness (more than one third missing). Further, 0.8% (n = 70) of the 24-hour recalls had to be excluded due to overreporting (>1,000 g of fruit and vegetables per day).

Results

24-Hour Recalls

The results of actual fruit and vegetable intakes (g/day) of all countries and the total group are presented in table 3.

Table 3. 24-Hour recall data

a Fruit and fruit juice intake (g/day) of CSS mothers by country

Country	n	Fruits						Fruit juice					
		mean	median	P10	P25	P75	P90	mean	median	P10	P25	P75	P90
Austria	1,255	188 (179–196)	150	0	100	300	400	245 (228–263)	200	0	0	400	600
Belgium	1,049	161 (152–169)	150	0	50	250	350	124 (112–136)	0	0	0	200	400
Denmark	1,238	203 (195–212)	200	0	100	300	400	88 (79–97)	0	0	0	200	300
Iceland	824	97 (89–104)	100	0	0	150	250	104 (92–116)	0	0	0	200	400
Netherlands	808	152 (143–160)	113	0	100	200	300	203 (187–220)	200	0	0	400	400
Norway	831	150 (141–159)	100	0	0	200	300	112 (100–125)	0	0	0	200	400
Portugal	1,346	211 (204–218)	200	50	100	300	400	103 (94–112)	0	0	0	200	400
Spain	759	176 (166–187)	150	0	100	250	350	179 (164–193)	200	0	0	300	400
Sweden	960	194 (185–203)	200	0	100	300	400	140 (127–153)	0	0	0	200	400
Total	9,070	175 (172–178)	150	0	100	250	350	143 (139–148)	0	0	0	200	400

b Vegetable and total fruit and vegetable intake (g/day) of CSS mothers by country

Country	n	Total vegetables						Total fruit and vegetables without juice					
		mean	median	P10	P25	P75	P90	mean	median	P10	P25	P75	P90
Austria	1,255	96 (91–102)	80	0	40	140	220	284 (274–295)	255	60	150	390	540
Belgium	1,049	150 (143–157)	140	28	60	210	300	311 (299–323)	290	60	160	430	575
Denmark	1,238	139 (132–146)	120	0	50	200	301	342 (331–354)	324	99	189	470	626
Iceland	824	91 (84–97)	65	0	20	131	214	188 (177–198)	155	5	80	264	390
Netherlands	808	112 (106–118)	100	40	60	140	220	264 (252–275)	240	60	160	360	480
Norway	831	95 (89–101)	70	0	40	140	205	245 (233–257)	220	50	105	340	475
Portugal	1,346	169 (163–175)	160	30	80	240	320	380 (370–390)	365	140	250	500	640
Spain	759	88 (82–94)	80	0	20	130	200	264 (251–278)	240	50	140	360	500
Sweden	960	124 (118–131)	100	10	55	174	265	318 (306–330)	290	80	180	430	590
Total	9,070	122 (120–124)	100	0	45	178	265	297 (293–301)	270	60	153	410	560

Figures in parentheses indicate 95% CIs. P = Percentile.

Fruit

The highest fruit consumption was measured in Portugal, followed by Denmark and Sweden (fig. 1). The lowest consumption was reported in Iceland and Norway (median 100 g/day). However, the proportion of nonconsumers was much higher in Iceland than in Norway. The nonconsumer rate of the total group was 18%. The lowest rate was observed in Portugal with only 8%, the highest in Iceland (37%).

Juice

The highest intake levels of fruit juice were observed in Austria, the Netherlands and Spain. In all other countries, more than half of the participants had not consumed any fruit juice on the day in question. The highest percentages of zero consumption were found in Denmark (69%) and Portugal (66%).

Vegetables

Portugal also achieved the highest consumption level of vegetables, followed by Belgium and Denmark. Spain was the country with the lowest average intake level. About a fifth of the Spanish mothers did not eat vegetables on the day in question, which was also observed in Norway, Iceland and Austria. The lowest rate of nonconsumers was found in the Dutch sample (7%).

Differences between countries were not only observed regarding total amounts, but also in the preferential composition of raw versus cooked vegetables (fig. 2). More than 2/3 of the total amount was eaten as cooked vegeta-

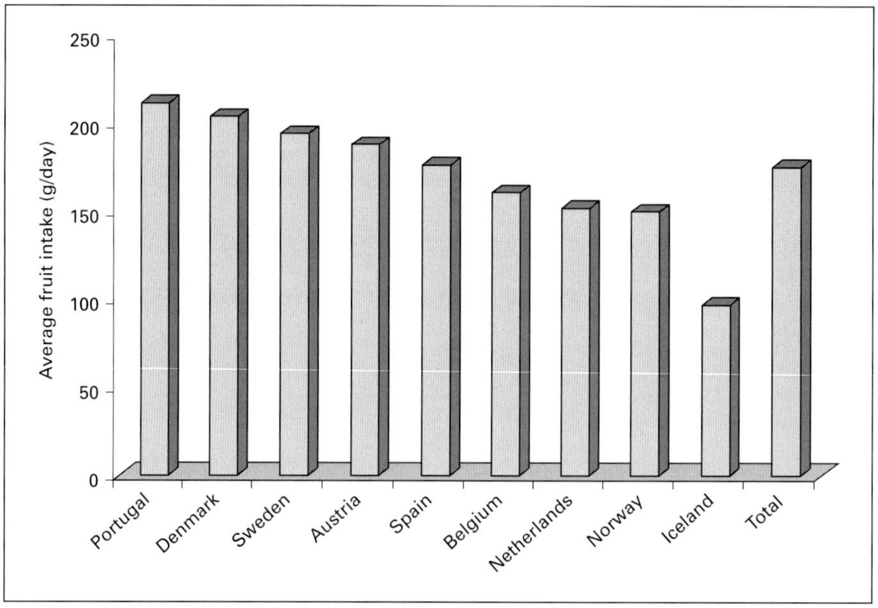

Fig. 1. Fruit consumption of CSS mothers by country (n = 9,070).

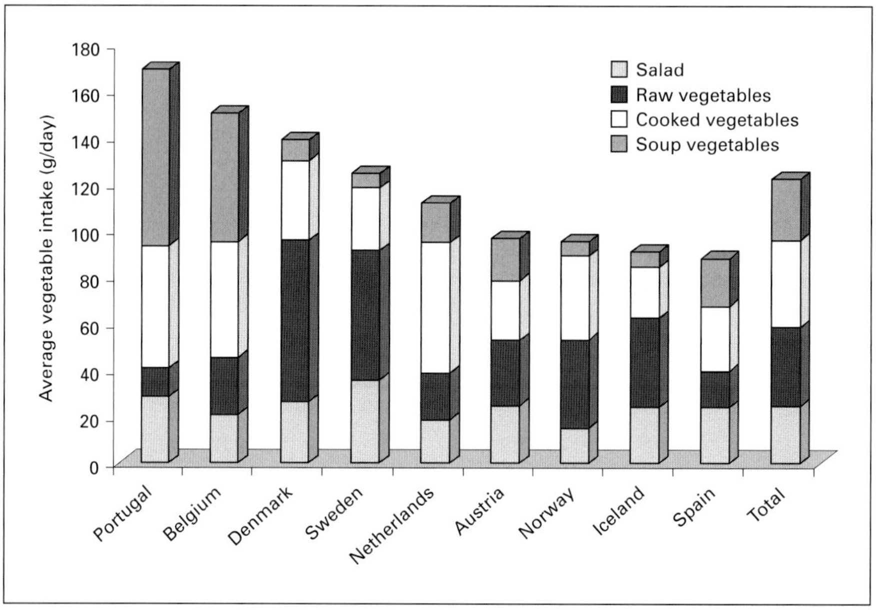

Fig. 2. Vegetable consumption of CSS mothers by country (n = 9,070).

bles in Portugal (76% of total vegetables), Belgium (70%) and the Netherlands (66%). Portugal and Belgium were additionally characterized by a high intake of vegetable soup. In contrast, a high consumption level of raw vegetables was observed in Sweden (73%), Denmark (69%) and Iceland (69%).

Overall, the WHO population goal of an average fruit and vegetable intake of at least 400 g/day was achieved in nearly every country (excepting Norway 357 g/day and Iceland 292 g/day) if fruit juice was included. When fruit juice was excluded, average consumption levels did not reach the recommendations in any country. The consumption levels were satisfying for only 27% of all participating mothers (table 4).

Food Frequency Questionnaire

The mean frequencies were '5–6 days per week' for fruit and 'once a day' for vegetables; 64% of the women indicated to eat vegetables every day, and daily fruit consumption was reported by 52%. Approximately 4.6%

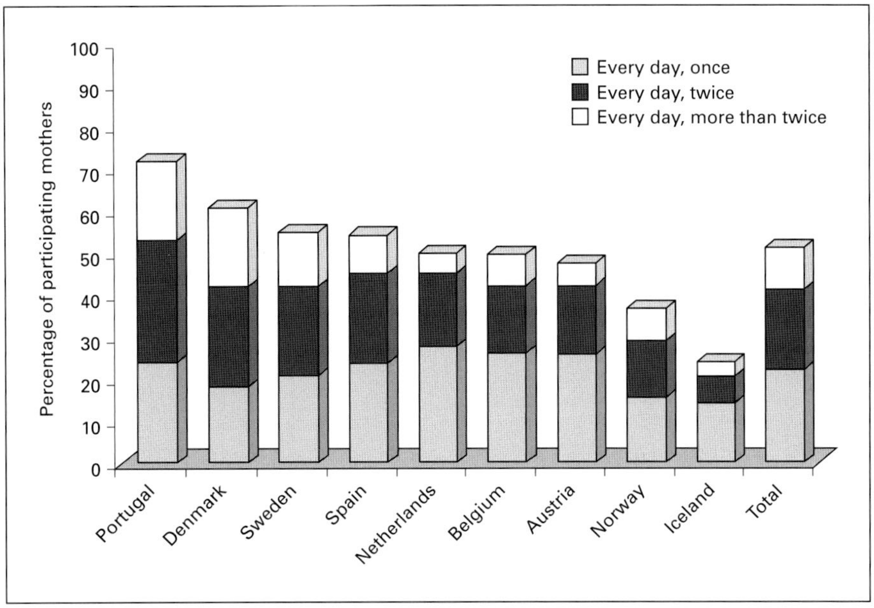

Fig. 3. Fruit consumption frequency of CSS mothers by country (n = 9,167).

Table 4. Percentage of mothers meeting WHO recommendations of ≥400 g/day

	Satisfying consumption of fruit and vegetables			
	≥400g/day without juice		≥400g/day including juice	
	n	% of participants	n	% of participants
Portugal	594	44.1	771	57.3
Denmark	440	35.5	613	49.5
Sweden	292	30.4	521	54.3
Belgium	308	29.4	503	48.0
Austria	292	23.3	705	56.2
Spain	156	20.6	389	51.3
Netherlands	150	18.6	447	55.3
Norway	147	17.7	319	38.4
Iceland	76	9.2	228	27.7
Total	2,455	27.1	4,496	49.6

(n = 422) of the total group were identified as nonconsumers (less than once a week) for fruit and 1.8% (n = 169) for vegetables. Iceland had the highest proportion of nonconsumers for fruit (8.3%). The highest rate of zero consumption of vegetables was found in Spain (4.1%), followed by Iceland (3.5%).

The highest percentage of daily fruit consumers was observed in Portugal, followed by Denmark, Sweden and Spain (fig. 3). Spain and Sweden had the highest intake frequencies of fruit juice. Portuguese mothers showed the highest rate in daily fruit consumption, but a low rate for fruit juice (11%). Austrian mothers had high daily juice intakes (18%), but were below the European average in the consumption of fresh fruit.

Daily vegetable consumption is illustrated in figure 4. The highest proportions of daily vegetable intake were found in Sweden, Belgium and Portugal. The lowest rates of daily vegetable consumers could be identified in Austria (52%) and Spain (51%).

Discussion

The present study shows that intake levels of fruit and vegetables are still below recommendations across Europe. In all participating countries, the consumption of vegetables is consistently lower than fruit. Since fruit intake is rather satisfactory across Europe, vegetable intake became the decisive factor in determining satisfactory levels for the total intake of both.

It is important to emphasize that the survey took place during a part of the year when local fruits and vegetables were highly available throughout Europe. Data collection during other times of the year might have shown even lower intakes for these special kinds of fruits and vegetables. The study did not include data on po-

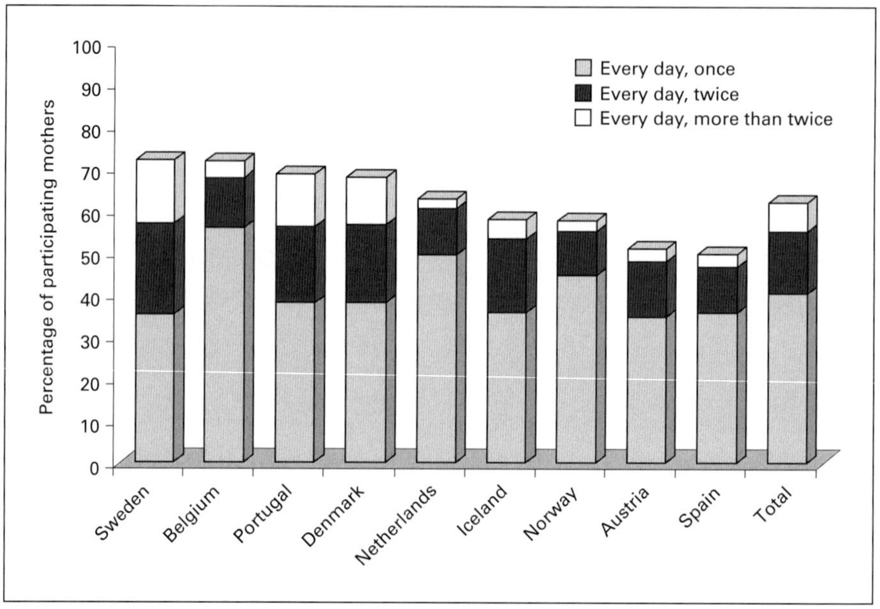

Fig. 4. Vegetable consumption frequency of CSS mothers by country (n = 9,167).

tato consumption, which in some countries contribute substantially to the intake of important vitamins, for example vitamin C and folate. Fruit juice as possible contributor to these vitamins was included and interpreted separately.

However, the intake quality and the vast differences in active compound content in different fruits and vegetables will be discussed in another paper. This paper mainly provides information about the crude amount of fruit and vegetable intake across Europe.

The comparison of intake levels in portions/day showed acceptable consumption levels for fruit in most participating countries. The WHO population goal of ≥400 g of fruit and vegetables per day represents 'the population average that is judged to be consistent with the maintenance of health'. The recommendation does not specify if fruit juice is considered as a part of total fruit consumption. Including fruit juice, the WHO population goal of ≥400 g/day was met by most surveyed countries, with the exception of Norway and Iceland. On the other hand, when fruit juice was excluded, average consumption did not reach the recommendations in any country.

Many national recommendations do not specify if they constitute minimum intake levels used as measurements in nutritional surveys or if they were designed for promoting desirable fruit and vegetable intakes among different target groups. There were also differences in the definition of food groups regarding inclusion of fruit juice, potatoes or tubers. For international comparisons, it would be desirable to have uniform guidelines designed for evaluation purpose.

For nutritional surveys, it is important to compare absolute amounts, but this is only possible to a limited extent, as exact portion sizes can only be provided by weighed protocols for several days including weekends, or repeated 24-hour recalls. All other instruments are more or less appropriate to show intake levels in grams. The precoded 24-hour recall used in the Pro Children study was also subject to the above limitation. Available information about 'portions' and 'pieces' had to be translated into standardized portion sizes in grams. In the Pro Children study, only weekday intakes were investigated.

The analysis of actual compared to usual intake showed coherence by country. This is particularly true for the ranking of countries according to their level of fruit intake. Both instruments showed high intakes in Portugal, Denmark and Sweden and very low ones in Iceland. High actual and usual vegetable intake levels were indicated in Portugal and Belgium. Sweden showed a high level of usual intake, but this could not be verified by the actual intake data. The low vegetable intake in Spain was again confirmed by both methods.

A south-north gradient of fruit and vegetable intake has been shown in several studies. This gradient is also reflected in different agricultural statistics [20] but could not be found in mothers of 11-year-old children participating in the Pro Children study.

Pro Children was not primarily designed to investigate fruit and vegetable consumption of European women in general. Considering the relatively high response rate, the study is representative of mothers of 11-year-old children in different regions of Europe. This study is the first to present such cross-national data of mothers collected with the same self-administered instrument. The data provide important information about fruit and vegetable consumption of mothers.

Conclusion

Fruit and vegetable intake levels are low in mothers of 11-year-olds across Europe. Despite the fact that Portugal and Denmark showed the highest consumptions of fruit and vegetables with an average intake without juice of 380 and 342 g/day, respectively, European mothers are far from meeting international recommendations. Especially vegetable consumption can be regarded as marginal in most of the surveyed countries. A high percentage of mothers indicated to eat fruit and vegetables less than once a day.

The results show that national and international interventions are necessary to promote fruit and especially vegetable consumption in the European population of mothers. A future paper will analyze the mother's intake versus the child's intake, which will provide additional information for these interventions.

Acknowledgements

This study is being carried out with financial support from the Commission of the European Communities, specific RTD program 'Quality of Life and Management of Living Resources', QLK1-2001-00547 'Promoting and Sustaining Health through Increased Fruit and Vegetable Consumption among European Schoolchildren' (Pro Children). The study does not necessarily reflect the Commission's views and in no way anticipates the Commission's future policy in this area. Special thanks to all mothers who took the time to participate in the Pro Children survey, to all people who were involved in data collection (e.g. headmasters, teachers and children) and finally to the staff and students from all 9 participating countries who coordinated the survey and entered the data.

References

1 Agudo A, Slimani N, Ocke MC, Naska A, Miller AB, Kroke A, et al: Consumption of vegetables, fruit and other plant foods in the European Prospective Investigation into Cancer and Nutrition (EPIC) cohorts from 10 European countries. Public Health Nutr 2002;5:1179–1196.

2 Trichopoulou A, Naska A, Antoniou A, Friel S, Trygg K, Turrini A: Vegetable and fruit: the evidence in their favour and the public health perspective. Int J Vitam Nutr Res 2003;73:63–69.

3 van't Veer P, Jansen MC, Klerk M, Kok FJ: Fruits and vegetables in the prevention of cancer and cardiovascular disease. Public Health Nutr 2000;3:103–107.

4 Thorsdottir I, Ramel A: Dietary intake of 10- to 16-year-old children and adolescents in central and northern Europe and association with the incidence of type 1 diabetes. Ann Nutr Metab 2003;47:267–275.

5 Nutrition and Diet for Healthy Lifestyles in Europe: Science and Policy Implications. Proceedings of the European Conference. May 18–20, 2000. Crete, Greece. Public Health Nutr 2001;4:337–434.

6 Food-based Dietary Guidelines in WHO European Member States. Copenhagen, WHO Regional Office for Europe, 2002.

7 WHO Global Strategy on Diet, Physical Activity and Health – what are the challenges for follow-up in Europe? Workshop 1. Eur J Public Health 2004;14(suppl 1):8.

8 Glade MJ: Food, nutrition, and the prevention of cancer: a global perspective. American Institute for Cancer Research/World Cancer Research Fund, American Institute for Cancer Research, 1997. Nutrition 1999;15:523–526.

9 Deutsche Gesellschaft für Ernährung, Österreichische Gesellschaft für Ernährung, Schweizerische Gesellschaft für Ernährungsforschung, Schweizerische Vereinigung für Ernährung: Referenzwerte für die Nährstoffzufuhr. Frankfurt, Umschau Braus GmbH, 2000.

10 Trolle E, Fagt S, Ovesen L: Fruit and vegetables, recommendations for intake; in: Danish Veterinary and Food Administration C. Copenhagen, Quickly Tryk A/S, 1998.

11 Steingrimsdottir L, Thorgeirsdottir H, Olafsdottir AS: The Diet of Icelanders; Dietary Survey of the Icelandic Nutrition Council 2002, Main findings: Icelandic Nutrition Council, 2003.

12 Zo eet Nederland. Den Haag, Voedingscentrum, 1998.

13 Blomhoff R, Lande B, Ose T: Recommendations for increased intake of fruit and vegetables: National Nutrition Council, Oslo. 1996.

14 Conselho Nacional de Alimentação e Nutrição. Comissão de Educação Alimentar. Recomendações para a educação alimentar da população portuguesa. Lisboa. Revista Portuguesa de Nutrição 1997;7:5–19.

15 Aranceta J, Serra-Majem L: Dietary guidelines for the Spanish population. Public Health Nutr 2001;4:1403–1408.

16 Statens Livsmedelsverk. Kost och motionsrekommendationer. Livsmedelsverket, Uppsala. 2004.

17 Steingrimsdottir L, Ovesen L, Moreiras O, Jacob S: Selection of relevant dietary indicators for health. Eur J Clin Nutr 2002;56:S8–S11.

18 Vasdeki VG, Stylianou S, Naska A: Estimation of age- and gender-specific food availability from household budget survey data. Public Health Nutr 2001;4:1149–1151.

19 Roos G, Johansson L, Kasmel A, Klumbiene J, Prattala R: Disparities in vegetable and fruit consumption: European cases from the north to the south. Public Health Nutr 2001;4:35–43.

20 Elmadfa I, Weichselbaum E, Koenig J, Remaut De Winter A-M, Trolle E, Haapala I, et al: European nutrition and health report 2004. Annals of Nutrition and Metabolism 2004, p 46.

21 Agudo A, Slimani N, Ocke MC, Naska A: Vegetable and fruit consumption in the EPIC cohorts from 10 European countries. IARC Sci Publ 2002;156:99–103.
22 Slimani N, Fahey M, Welch AA, Wirfalt E, Stripp C, Bergstrom E, et al: Diversity of dietary patterns observed in the European Prospective Investigation into Cancer and Nutrition (EPIC) project. Public Health Nutr 2002; 5:1311–1328.
23 Kvaavik E, Meyer HE, Selmer RM, Egeland G, Tverdal A: [Food habits in Hedmark related to gender, education and marital status]. Tidsskr Nor Laegeforen 1999;119:3406–3409.
24 Hjartaker A, Lund E: Relationship between dietary habits, age, lifestyle, and socio-economic status among adult Norwegian women. The Norwegian Women and Cancer Study. Eur J Clin Nutr 1998;52:565–572.
25 Tur JA, Romaguera D, Pons A: Food consumption patterns in a mediterranean region: does the mediterranean diet still exist? Ann Nutr Metab 2004;48:193–201.
26 Sanchez-Villegas A, De Irala J, Martinez-Gonzalez MA: [The Mediterranean diet and cardiovascular disease: results of a pilot study from the SUN project (University of Navarre Follow-Up Study)]. Rev Med Univ Navarra 2002;46:9–16.
27 Aranceta J, Perez Rodrigo C, Eguileor I, Marzana I, Gonzalez de Galdeano L, Saenz de Buruaga J: Food consumption patterns in the adult population of the Basque Country (EINUT-I). Public Health Nutr 1998;1:185–192.
28 Reis MF, Oliveira L, Pereirinha A, Pereira Miguel JM: Fruit and vegetable intake and chronic disease risk in Portugal. IARC Sci Publ 2002;156:137–138.
29 Elmadfa I, Freisling H, Koenig J, Blachfelner J, Cvitkovich-Steiner H, Genser D, et al: Austrian Nutrition Report 2003. Vienna: Institute of Nutritional Sciences, University of Vienna, Cooperation with the Federal Ministry of Health and Women, 2003.
30 Lassen A, Thorsen AV, Trolle E, Elsig M, Ovesen L: Successful strategies to increase the consumption of fruits and vegetables: results from the Danish '6 a day' Work-site Canteen Model Study. Public Health Nutr 2004;7:263–270.
31 Haraldsdottir J, Astrup AV, Dynesen AW, Holm L: [Steadily changing food consumption of Danes. Clear trends during the period 1995–2001]. Ugeskr Laeger 2002;164:2028–2033.
32 Lowik MR, Hulshof KF, Brussaard JH: Patterns of food and nutrient intakes of Dutch adults according to intakes of total fat, saturated fatty acids, dietary fibre, and of fruit and vegetables. Br J Nutr 1999;81:S91–S98.
33 Lindstrom M, Hanson BS, Wirfalt E, Ostergren PO: Socioeconomic differences in the consumption of vegetables, fruit and fruit juices. The influence of psychosocial factors. Eur J Public Health 2001;11:51–59.
34 Becker W: Dietary guidelines and patterns of food and nutrient intake in Sweden. Br J Nutr 1999;81:S113–S117.
35 Becker W MP: Dietary habits and nutrient intake in Sweden 1997–1998. The 2nd National food consumption survey. English Summary. Livsmedelsverket, Uppsala. 2003.
36 De Henauw S, De Backer G: Nutrient and food intakes in selected subgroups of Belgian adults. Br J Nutr 1999;81:S37–S42.
37 Irala-Estevez JD, Groth M, Johansson L, Oltersdorf U, Prattala R, Martinez-Gonzalez MA: A systematic review of socio-economic differences in food habits in Europe: consumption of fruit and vegetables. Eur J Clin Nutr 2000;54:706–714.
38 Beer-Borst S, Hercberg S, Morabia A, Bernstein MS, Galan P, Galasso R, et al: Dietary patterns in six european populations: results from EURALIM, a collaborative European data harmonization and information campaign. Eur J Clin Nutr 2000;54:253–262.
39 Haraldsdóttir J, Thórsdóttir I, de Almeida MDV, Maes L, de Rodrigues C, Elmadfa I, Anderson LF: Validity and reproducibility of a precoded questionnaire to assess fruit and vegetable intake in European 11- to 12-year old schoolchildren. Ann Nutr Metab 2005;49:221–227.
40 Kristjansdottir A, Andersen L, Haraldsdóttir J, de Almeida MDV, Thórsdóttir I: Validity of a questionnaire to assess fruit and vegetable intake in adults. Eur J Clin Nutr, submitted.
41 Klepp K-I, Pérez-Rodrigo C, De Bourdeaudhuij I, Due P, Elmadfa I, Haraldsdóttir J, König J, Sjöström M, Thórsdóttir I, de Almeida MDV, Yngve A, Brug J: Promoting fruit and vegetable consumption among European schoolchildren: Rationale, conceptualization and design of the Pro Children Project. Ann Nutr Metab 2005;49:212–220.

Annals of
Nutrition& Metabolism

Ann Nutr Metab 2005;49:255–266
DOI: 10.1159/000087332

Published online: August 3, 2005

Personal, Social and Environmental Factors regarding Fruit and Vegetable Intake among Schoolchildren in Nine European Countries

The Pro Children Study

Camilla Sandvik[a,b] Ilse De Bourdeaudhuij[c] Pernille Due[d] Johannes Brug[e] Marianne Wind[e] Elling Bere[a] Carmen Pérez-Rodrigo[f] Alexandra Wolf[g] Ibrahim Elmadfa[g] Inga Thórsdóttir[h,i] Maria Daniel Vaz de Almeida[j] Agneta Yngve[k] Knut-Inge Klepp[a]

[a]Department of Nutrition, Faculty of Medicine, University of Oslo, Oslo and [b]Research Centre for Health Promotion, Department of Education and Health Promotion, Faculty of Psychology, University of Bergen, Bergen, Norway; [c]Department of Movement and Sport Sciences, Ghent University, Ghent, Belgium; [d]Department of Social Medicine, Institute of Public Health, Faculty of Health Sciences, University of Copenhagen, Copenhagen, Denmark; [e]Department of Public Health, Erasmus University Medical Centre, Rotterdam, The Netherlands; [f]Community Nutrition Unit of Bilbao, Bilbao, Spain; [g]Institute for Nutritional Sciences, University of Vienna, Vienna, Austria; [h]Unit for Nutrition Research, Landspitali University Hospital and [i]Department of Food Science, University of Iceland, Reykjavik, Iceland; [j]Faculty of Nutrition and Food Sciences, University of Porto, Porto, Portugal; [k]Unit for Preventive Nutrition, Department of Biosciences, Karolinska Institute, Stockholm, Sweden

Key Words

European schoolchildren · Psychosocial correlates · Environmental correlates · Fruit intake · Vegetable intake · Pro Children study

Abstract

Background/Aims: Children in Europe are consuming less fruit and vegetables than recommended. Knowledge about the potential determinants of fruit and vegetable intake is vital to understand discrepancies in intake and to guide interventions. The aim of the present study was to assess personal, social and environmental factors regarding fruit and vegetable intake among 11- to 12-year-old children in Europe. ***Methods:*** A cross-sectional survey was undertaken, with nationally or regionally representative samples of in total 13,305 children (mean age 11.4 years) from nine European countries. Pupils in the classroom completed a self-administered questionnaire measuring fruit and vegetable intake and personal, social and environmental factors during one school lesson. Age-adjusted covariance analyses were carried out by gender, for the full sample and for each country separately. Proportions responding positively to the constructs are presented. ***Results:*** Overall, European children held a positive attitude towards fruit and vegetable intake. For some constructs, large between-country differences were found. Children had a more positive attitude towards fruit than towards vegetables, and girls were on average more positive than boys. The children perceived their social environment as supportive towards fruit and vegetable intake. They reported good to very good availability of fruit and vegetables at home. However, availability at school and during leisure time

KARGER

Fax +41 61 306 12 34
E-Mail karger@karger.ch
www.karger.com

0250–6807/05/0494–0255$22.00/0

Accessible online at:
www.karger.com/anm

Camilla Sandvik
Research Centre for Health Promotion, Department of Education and Health Promotion
Faculty of Psychology, University of Bergen, PO Box 7800
NO–5020 Bergen (Norway)
Tel. +47 55 58 47 99, Fax +47 55 58 98 87, E-Mail camilla.sandvik@iuh.uib.no

activities seemed to be low, both for fruit and for vegetables. ***Conclusion:*** A large majority of the children reported positively to the personal and social factors regarding fruit and vegetable intake. As regards availability of fruit and vegetables at school and leisure time, and accessibility of fruit and vegetables at home, there is room for improvement.

Introduction

Results from the Pro Children study show that the current fruit and vegetable intake levels are below recommendations for children across European countries [1]. Children are at an age when habits are learned. Moreover, eating habits in childhood may be strongly predictive of those in adulthood [2–4]. Interventions promoting fruit and vegetable intake in this age group are thus urgently needed. However, before designing adequate intervention programmes, information is needed about the factors that may influence fruit and vegetable intake [5]. No cross-national or cross-regional studies with a specific focus on fruit and vegetables using a single methodology in assessing consumption and its correlates among children or adolescents have been carried out in Europe [6]. Most of the published studies investigating factors associated with fruit and vegetable intake among children and adolescents have been conducted in the USA [see for instance, 7–10]. The relatively few European studies that have been undertaken report data from single countries and often focus on a restricted number of possible correlates [6]. Thus, there is a lack of international, comparative studies investigating potential determinants of fruit and vegetable intake. Furthermore, there is a need to apply theory in a more systematic manner when investigating these determinants [6, 11].

In the Pro Children study, constructs from different behavioural theories were included to ensure inclusion of a large range of potential determinants at the individual, social and environmental level [6]. Social cognitive theory, the ASE model, the Theory of Triadic influence, as well as a social-ecological perspective on health behaviour were used to develop the theoretical framework for the study [6].

The present study is the first to report on differences in potential personal, social and environmental determinants of fruit and vegetable intake among 11- to 12-year-old children between the nine different Pro Children countries (Austria, Belgium, Denmark, Iceland, the Netherlands, Norway, Portugal, Spain and Sweden).

Methods

Sample and Procedure

A cross-sectional study was carried out, with nationally representative samples drawn in each country (except for Austria, where the sample was representative for the eastern region, covering 42% of the total population, and Belgium, where the sample was representative for Flanders only), aiming for at least 1,300 schoolchildren from each country. The full sample consisted of 14,147 schoolchildren from the nine Pro Children countries. Of the 13,924 questionnaires returned, 110 were unanswered and 144 were destroyed on parents' request. Research centres excluded 306 questionnaires because they were judged unreliable, and 59 questionnaires were excluded because gender information was missing. This left us with 13,305 completed questionnaires for analyses. Mean age was 11.4 years (range 8.8–13.8), with the large majority (79%) of the children born in 1992. Final sample sizes varied from 1,105 for the Netherlands to 2,134 for Portugal. Total response rate was 90.4%. Gender distribution was fairly equal for all countries, with Spain, Belgium and the Netherlands having the largest gender discrepancy (46% girls and 54% boys for Spain and Belgium; the reverse pattern for the Netherlands; table 1).

Data were collected in all countries from October to early December 2003. The survey questionnaires were mailed to the participating schools. The pupils completed the questionnaires in the classroom during one school lesson (45 min). The Pro Children Project adheres to the Helsinki Declaration and the conventions of the Council of Europe on human rights and biomedicine. Ethical approval and research clearance was obtained from the relevant ethics committees in all countries where this applied. Research permission was obtained from national and local school authorities (local school boards and headmasters) and from national and local school health authorities before parents and students were contacted. All students and their parents received written information on the project prior to data collection, completion of the questionnaires was voluntary and parents could demand that their child's questionnaire not be used in the study.

Questionnaire

An elaborate description of the development, reliability and validity of the determinant part of the questionnaire has been published by De Bourdeaudhuij et al. [12]. In short, the questionnaire was a self-administered teacher-guided instrument, based on the Pro Children theoretical framework. The questionnaire included questions on fruit and vegetable consumption as well as psychosocial factors. The same psychosocial constructs as presented in De Bourdeaudhuij et al. [12] are used in this paper, with one exception: 'parental facilitation' has been added. This is measured by one item: 'Does your mother or father usually cut up fruit/vegetables for you in between meals?' with response categories measured on a 5-point scale, going from 1 = yes, always to 5 = never (see Appendix for an overview of the items, constructs and scaling).

Statistical Analyses

To compute scales for the constructs, all items were recoded from –2 to +2. Scales were made by calculating the mean from the relevant item scores. Respondents who answered fewer than half of the relevant items for a given scale were given a missing value for that scale. Thus, the number of children included in each analysis varies according to the number of pupils who have replied to at least half the items for that specific construct. All items were coded in the same direction, so that a higher score implied more agreement with the statement. 'Perceived barriers' are also coded like this, so that a higher score on perceived barriers means higher agreement with barriers against eating fruit or vegetables. As recommended [11], Cronbach's alpha analyses were run for all scales for the full sample. As for the test-retest sample [12], Cronbach's alphas were somewhat higher for the vegetable scales than for fruit (see Appendix). In general, internal consistency results were similar to the ones reported for the test-retest study.

To present the proportions of children answering positively to the psychosocial factors regarding fruit and vegetable intake, the score for each scale was dichotomized. Arbitrarily, we used +0.5 (instead of 0) as the cut-off point for a positive construct, to distinguish it from negative as well as neutral. All values from –2 to 0.49 were given the value 0 (negative to neutral) and all values from 0.5 to 2 the value 1 (positive). Since higher scores for 'perceived barriers' mean stronger perceived barriers against eating fruit or vegetable, for this construct, a cut-off of –0.5 was used. Age-adjusted, univariate analyses of covariance were carried out for each construct by gender, for the full sample and for each country separately. Because of the large sample size, 99% confidence intervals are presented for the full sample and 95% confidence intervals are used for within-country comparison. Results are discussed in terms of differences believed to be of practical importance, and not only in terms of statistical significance. Consequently, country differences are presented and discussed when a country differs 20 percentage points or more from the proportion for all countries. Gender differences within countries are presented and discussed when the difference is 10 percentage points or more. Since fruit and vegetable intake are multidetermined behaviours [13] and determinants of fruit intake may differ from determinants of vegetable intake [14, 15], analyses were done separately for factors regarding fruit and for vegetable intake. Data were analysed using SPSS 12.0.01.

Results

Fruit

Personal Factors

More than 80% of the children reported a positive attitude towards eating fruit, and a high confidence (self-efficacy) that they can eat fruit if they decide to do so. Approximately 90% of the children said they like to eat fruit and reported a strong preference for different kinds of fruit. Three quarters of the children reported an intention to eat fruit every day, and few said that they experienced barriers such as wanting to eat something else instead as a reason for any lack of fruit consumption. Overall, 45% thought they ate much or very much fruit and about 60% reported that eating fruit is a habit for them. In general, knowledge about recommended intake levels was low, as only 58% of the sample knew that they should eat at least two pieces of fruit every day. For all these constructs, girls were more positive than boys (table 2).

For most personal constructs, we found small differences between countries in the proportions of children who had a positive attitude to fruit. The largest differences were found for knowledge about the national recommendation. In Belgium, only 45% of the children knew that they should eat at least two pieces of fruit per day, while in Portugal about 70% reported the correct recommendation. Furthermore, Spanish children reported low self-efficacy levels, and a smaller proportion of Belgian children answered positively to the intention and habit questions compared to the full sample. Gender differences were large in all the Nordic countries for self-rated in-

Table 1. Characteristics of sample

	Countries									
	All	Austria	Belgium	Denmark	Iceland	Netherlands	Norway	Portugal	Spain	Sweden
Sample size	13,305	1,692	1,343	1,919	1,196	1,105	1,196	2,134	1,313	1,407
Boys	6,680 (50.2)	805 (47.6)	728 (54.2)	978 (51.0)	629 (52.6)	511 (46.2)	607 (50.8)	1,012 (47.4)	705 (53.7)	705 (50.1)
Age (mean ± SD), years	11.4±0.48	11.0±0.59	11.5±0.46	11.4±0.38	11.3±0.33	11.7±0.46	11.3±0.30	11.5±0.45	11.4±0.44	1.4±0.47
Age range	8.8–13.8	8.8–13.5	10.3–13.8	9.5–13.2	9.8–12.1	10.3–13.6	10.4–13.4	10.8–12.8	9.8–13.8	9.8–13.6
Number of classes/ schools	723 classes/ 375 schools	73 classes/ 23 schools	73 classes/ 50 schools	105 classes/ 59 schools	68 classes/ 32 schools	62 classes/ 49 schools	73 classes/ 52 schools	128 classes/ 27 schools	64 classes/ 37 schools	77 classes/ 46 schools
Response rate	90.4%	95.3%	84.5%	92.0%	88.7%	79.7%	89.5%	98.4%	94.7%	84.2%

Note that response rate is the number of students' questionnaires returned, in relation to total number of students in participating classes. Thus, attrition consists of students being absent on the day the survey was carried out, as well as students present but denying to participate, or not being allowed to participate by their parents. Figures in parentheses indicate percentages.

take, with a higher proportion of girls reporting positively on fruit intake than boys. For intention to eat fruit, there were substantial gender differences for Belgium, Denmark and Iceland, whereas for habit, substantial gender differences were found in all countries, except Austria and Spain (table 2).

Social Factors

Overall, two thirds of the children reported that their parents or best friends eat fruit every day, and more than half the sample reported that their parents encourage them to eat fruit every day. About 40% answered that their parents demand that they eat fruit every day, whereas almost 90% indicated that their parents allowed them to eat fruit every day. However, only 27% reported that their parents facilitate fruit consumption by cutting up fruit for them on most days or always. Overall, there was a higher proportion of girls who answered positively on all social constructs, except parental facilitation. Differences between countries were somewhat larger for the social-environmental factors, indicating a north-south gradient. A higher proportion of children in the southern countries (Portugal and Spain) reported positive role model behaviour, active parental encouragement and parental demands to eat fruit. In the Nordic countries (Norway and Sweden) but also in Belgium, a low proportion of the children reported that their parents demand that they eat fruit every day, and in Denmark, active parental encouragement was clearly lower than in the other countries. Also for parental facilitation, we found marked country differences, with more than 40% of the Austrian children and of Portuguese boys reporting that their parents cut fruit for them, while this was reported by only 10% of the Norwegian boys. No clear pattern of gender differences within countries were

Table 2. Proportion (%), with confidence intervals in parentheses, of boys/girls reporting positively on constructs related to fruit intake in children: The Pro Children Study

Constructs	Countries									
	All		Austria		Belgium		Denmark		Iceland	
	M	F	M	F	M	F	M	F	M	F
Personal										
Self-rated intake	43.9 (42.3–45.5)	49.0 (47.5–50.6)	52.8 (49.3–56.2)	58.6 (55.3–61.9)	41.2 (37.6–44.8)	45.2 (41.3–49.1)	43.9 (40.7–47.1)	52.5 (49.3–55.7)	32.8 (28.9–36.6)	42.7 (38.7–46.7)
Knowledge	55.0 (53.4–56.5)	60.5 (58.9–62.0)	60.7 (60.5–67.0)	63.8 (60.5–67.0)	42.2 (38.6–45.8)	47,3 (43.4–51.2)	64.1 (61.1–67.2)	66.8 (63.8–69.9)	50.2 (46.3–54.2)	56.3 (52.2–60.5)
Attitudes	85.2 (84.1–86.3)	88.7 (87.6–89.8)	89.9 (88.0–91.9)	92.2 (90.3–94.0)	79.7 (76.7–82.7)	77.6 (74.3–80.8)	79.0 (76.5–81.4)	85.7 (83.2–88.1)	81.7 (78.9–84.5)	89.0 (86.1–91.9)
Liking	89.4 (88.5–90.3)	93.9 (93.0–94.8)	90.2 (88.3–92.1)	94.0 (92.2–95.7)	86.1 (83.8–88.4)	91.8 (89.3–94.3)	87.4 (85.5–89.2)	94.3 (92.4–96.2)	91.0 (89.2–92.8)	98.1 (96.2–99.9)
General self-efficacy	79.8 (78.6–81.1)	83.0 (81.7–84.2)	83.4 (80.8–86.0)	83.0 (80.5–85.5)	73.6 (70.5–76.6)	81.7 (78.4–85.0)	80.9 (78.5–83.3)	83.6 (81.2–86.1)	78.8 (75.9–81.7)	88.2 (85.1–91.3)
Intention	73.6 (72.3–74.9)	81.6 (80.2–82.9)	78.6 (75.9–81.4)	82.0 (79.4–84.6)	60.4 (57.0–63.9)	71.6 (67.8–75.3)	73.3 (70.8–75.9)	84.3 (81.7–86.9)	75.9 (72.8–79.0)	86.7 (83.4–89.9)
Habit	56.8 (55.2–58.3)	65.3 (63.7–6.8)	67.0 (63.8–70.3)	71.0 (67.9–74.0)	41.8 (38.1–45.4)	49.5 (45.6–53.5)	53.0 (49.8–56.1)	65.1 (61.9–68.2)	50.9 (47.0–54.8)	61.5 (57.4–65.6)
Preferences	87.0 (86.0–88.0)	91.9 (90.9–92.9)	91.6 (89.9–93.4)	94.6 (93.0–96.3)	84.9 (82.6–87.2)	93.3 (90.8–95.8)	85.1 (83.0–87.2)	91.0 (88.9–93.1)	87.1 (84.7–89.4)	93.8 (91.3–96.3)
Perceived barriers	13.1 (12.1–14.1)	7.8 (6.8–8.8)	15.9 (13.6–18.2)	9.2 (7.0–11.3)	13.3 (11.1–15.5)	7.3 (4.9–9.7)	13.2 (11.3–15.2)	7.7 (5.7–9.6)	10.9 (8.7–13.0)	4.6 (2.4–6.8)
Perceived social env ironment										
Subjective norm/ modelling	61.3 (59.8–62.8)	67.6 (66.1–69.1)	76.9 (74.0–79.9)	77.5 (74.7–80.3)	44.5 (40.9–48.2)	49.9 (46.0–53.9)	48.0 (44.8–51.2)	56.7 (53.5–59.9)	50.4 (46.5–54.3)	57.4 (53.3–61.5)
Active parental encouragement	55.7 (54.1–57.3)	59.5 (58.0–61.1)	59.5 (56.1–62.9)	61.3 (58.0–64.5)	53.2 (49.5–56.8)	51.9 (47.9–55.9)	35.5 (32.5–38.6)	35.9 (32.8–39.0)	57.4 (53.6–61.3)	65.0 (60.9–69.0)
Demand family rule	39.7 (38.1–41.3)	44.0 (42.4–45.6)	31.6 (28.3–34.9)	31.2 (28.1–34.3)	25.1 (21.9–28.3)	25.9 (22.4–29.4)	34.4 (31.3–37.5)	33.8 (30.7–36.9)	37.7 (33.7–41.7)	47.2 (43.0–51.3)
Allow family rule	86.7 (85.6–87.8)	88.6 (87.5–89.6)	94.5 (93.0–96.0)	96.3 (94.9–97.7)	85.4 (82.7–88.0)	84.9 (82.0–87.7)	87.9 (85.8–90.0)	89.5 (87.4–91.6)	89.0 (86.6–91.4)	91.7 (89.2–94.2)
Parental facilitation	27.4 (26.0–28.9)	26.5 (25.1–27.9)	41.3 (37.9–44.8)	43.5 (40.2–46.8)	25.6 (22.4–28.8)	26.0 (22.5–29.4)	20.4 (17.8–23.0)	19.1 (16.5–21.7)	21.6 (18.4–24.8)	18.8 (15.5–22.2)
Perceived physical environment										
Availability at home	88.1 (87.1–89.0)	90.7 (89.7–91.7)	93.6 (91.9–95.3)	94.0 (92.4–95.6)	84.9 (82.4–87.3)	88.4 (85.7–91.1)	88.6 (86.5–90.6)	89.0 (86.9–91.0)	76.0 (72.8–79.2)	82.8 (79.4–86.1)
Availability at school and leisure	21.5 (20.1–22.8)	23.2 (21.8–24.5)	43.6 (40.1–47.1)	46.9 (43.6–50.3)	17.3 (14.5–20.2)	20.1 (17.0–23.2)	35.8 (32.7–39.0)	33.7 (30.6–36.9)	9.2 (6.9–11.4)	8.6 (6.2–11.0)

found for the social factors. We did observe, however, that a substantially higher proportion of girls in Norway reported positively on active parental encouragement, whereas a substantially higher proportion of girls than boys in the Netherlands and Iceland reported parental demand to eat fruit (table 2).

Environmental Factors

About 90% of the children reported that fruit is available at home always or on most days. However, both boys and girls reported much lower availability of fruit at school and leisure time activities. Only 22% said that they can get fruit at school, at their friends' house and at places where they have their leisure time activities. Almost half of the children in the total sample said they can never get fruit at school, 8% said they can never get it at their friends' house, whereas 32% said they can never get fruit at the place of their leisure time activities (results not shown in table 2). There were almost no country differences in the proportions of children who reported fruit to be available at home, except for Icelandic boys, who were less likely to report a positive home availability than children from the other countries. Large between-country differences were found in availability at school and leisure time activities with a low of 5% of the Dutch children and a high of 45% of the Austrian children reporting fruit to be available at school and leisure time activities most days or always.

Vegetables

Personal Factors

About 70% of the children in the survey reported that they liked to eat vegetables, and about three quarters held a positive attitude towards vegetables. Around 60% reported a positive preference for different kinds of vegeta-

Table 2 (continued)

Constructs	Countries									
	Netherlands		Norway		Portugal		Spain		Sweden	
	M	F	M	F	M	F	M	F	M	F
Personal										
Self-rated intake	35.7 (31.4–39.9)	41.7 (37.7–45.6)	42.9 (38.8–47.0)	53.1 (49.0–57.2)	45.9 (42.9–49.0)	44.3 (41.4–47.2)	43.6 (39.9–47.3)	41.8 (37.8–45.8)	50.0 (46.4–53.7)	58.3 (54.6–62.0)
Knowledge	45.3 (40.9–49.6)	50.6 (46.6–54.7)	53.4 (49.3–57.5)	60.7 (56.6–64.8)	67.7 (64.9–70.5)	73.9 (71.2–76.5)	53.3 (49.6–57.1)	58.0 (54.0–62.0)	44.7 (41.0–48.4)	51.7 (48.0–55.4)
Attitudes	78.5 (74.9–82.0)	80.7 (77.5–84.0)	84.9 (82.2–87.6)	91.0 (88.3–93.6)	92.5 (91.0–93.9)	95.6 (94.2–97.0)	90.8 (88.7–92.8)	93.2 (91.0–95.4)	85.8 (83.3–88.3)	88.3 (85.8–90.8)
Liking	86.6 (83.8–89.4)	89.7 (87.1–92.3)	92.5 (90.7–94.3)	97.4 (95.6–99.1)	93.0 (91.6–94.5)	95.5 (94.2–96.9)	84.7 (82.2–87.2)	90.7 (88.0–93.3)	92.0 (90.0–94.0)	92.9 (91.0–94.9)
General self-efficacy	75.3 (71.6–79.0)	77.7 (74.3–81.2)	82.8 (79.9–85.7)	88.5 (85.7–91.4)	83.0 (80.8–85.3)	85.2 (83.1–87.4)	71.6 (68.2–75.0)	71.2 (67.5–74.8)	85.7 (83.1–88.3)	85.5 (82.8–88.1)
Intention	69.0 (65.1–72.9)	77.3 (73.7–80.8)	78.4 (75.3–81.6)	86.8 (83.7–89.9)	79.8 (77.4–82.2)	83.4 (81.1–85.6)	69.7 (66.4–73.0)	77.8 (74.2–81.3)	73.6 (70.6–76.7)	82.3 (79.2–85.4)
Habit	54.5 (50.1–58.8)	63.6 (59.6–67.6)	47.0 (42.9–51.0)	61.7 (57.7–65.8)	72.7 (70.0–75.4)	77.2 (74.7–79.7)	61.6 (58.0–65.3)	64.7 (60.8–68.6)	52.6 (48.9–56.2)	61.2 (57.5–64.8)
Preferences	79.5 (76.2–82.8)	85.8 (82.7–88.8)	87.8 (85.4–90.2)	94.1 (91.7–96.4)	90.7 (89.1–92.3)	94.8 (93.2–96.3)	81.2 (78.4–84.1)	85.4 (82.4–88.5)	91.0 (88.9–93.2)	92.0 (89.9–94.0)
Perceived barriers	10.3 (8.1–12.5)	4.0 (2.0–6.0)	11.8 (9.3–14.3)	8.2 (5.7–10.7)	14.9 (12.9–16.9)	9.8 (7.9–11.8)	17.6 (14.9–20.4)	13.9 (11.0–16.9)	7.1 (5.4–8.8)	3.9 (2.2–5.6)
Perceived social environment										
Subjective norm/ modelling	61.2 (57.0–65.3)	70.7 (66.9–74.5)	52.1 (48.0–56.2)	60.6 (56.5–64.6)	80.6 (78.2–83.0)	83.2 (80.9–85.4)	72.9 (69.7–76.1)	79.5 (76.1–83.0)	57.0 (53.3–60.7)	61.4 (57.7–65.1)
Active parental encouragement	46.9 (42.5–51.3)	50.3 (46.3–54.4)	44.0 (39.9–48.1)	54.5 (50.5–58.6)	77.3 (74.8–79.9)	78.5 (76.1–80.9)	72.2 (69.0–75.4)	79.5 (76.0–83.0)	48.4 (44.7–52.1)	55.5 (51.8–59.2)
Demand family rule	41.2 (36.8–45.6)	54.3 (50.3–58.3)	13.3 (10.2–16.3)	18.2 (15.2–21.2)	75.0 (72.3–77.7)	76.2 (73.6–78.7)	57.9 (54.2–61.6)	63.6 (59.6–67.5)	27.3 (23.9–30.7)	29.7 (26.3–33.1)
Allow family rule	85.4 (82.3–88.6)	84.5 (81.5–87.4)	84.2 (81.3–87.0)	88.0 (85.1–90.8)	86.6 (84.5–88.7)	88.1 (86.1–90.1)	78.4 (75.4–81.5)	82.3 (79.0–85.5)	86.5 (84.1–89.0)	88.9 (86.4–91.4)
Parental facilitation	30.1 (26.0–34.2)	32.2 (28.4–35.9)	10.3 (7.5–13.1)	15.3 (12.6–18.1)	41.6 (38.5–44.6)	32.5 (29.7–35.4)	29.3 (25.9–32.7)	28.5 (24.8–32.1)	17.6 (14.9–20.4)	15.0 (12.3–17.8)
Perceived physical environment										
Availability at home	88.3 (85.7–90.9)	91.9 (89.6–94.3)	82.7 (79.6–85.7)	85.9 (82.9–88.9)	92.3 (90.7–93.9)	94.0 (92.6–95.5)	91.5 (89.6–93.5)	94.2 (92.1–96.3)	89.9 (87.8–92.1)	91.6 (89.5–93.8)
Availability at school and leisure	4.7 (2.8–6.6)	5.1 (3.3–6.8)	12.1 (9.3–14.8)	12.1 (9.3-–14.9)	24.1 (21.4–26.9)	27.8 (25.2–30.3)	10.4 (8.1–12.8)	11.0 (8.5–13.5)	17.6 (14.5–20.7)	22.8 (19.7–25.9)

bles; about a third of the children thought they ate many or very many vegetables, and 1 in 5 thought they ate more vegetables than other children at their age. Concerning knowledge about recommended intake levels, 23% of the total sample correctly reported that they should eat three portions or serving spoons or more each day. About half of the children, girls more so than boys, expressed that they wanted to eat vegetables every day, while a smaller proportion reported that it was a habit for them to eat vegetables every day.

Between-country differences for liking vegetables were large. More than 80% of girls in Norway and Iceland reported positively on liking items, compared to slightly more than half the children in Spain. Spanish children also reported substantially lower than average on self-efficacy, and only one third reported an intention to eat vegetables. In contrast, more than 70% of Norwegian and Icelandic girls said they wanted to eat vegetables every day. Fewer Spanish children reported positively on habit and preferences, while a higher proportion reported experiencing barriers towards eating vegetables compared to the other children. For self-rated vegetable intake, liking, intention to eat vegetables and habit, substantial gender differences were seen in Norway only, with higher scores for girls than for boys.

Social Factors

About 60% of the children reported that their parents or best friends eat vegetables every day. More than half the sample reported that they were encouraged to eat vegetables by their parents, the numbers being slightly lower than for fruit. Only about one fourth of the children reported that their parents regularly cut up vegetables for them to eat in-between meals, with large between-country

Table 3. Proportion (%),with confidence intervals in parentheses, of boys/girls reporting positively on constructs related to vegetable intake in children: The Pro Children Study

Constructs	Countries									
	All		Austria		Belgium		Denmark		Iceland	
	M	F	M	F	M	F	M	F	M	F
Personal										
Self-rated intake	37.1 (35.5–38.6)	40.7 (39.2–42.3)	37.2 (33.8–40.6)	40.3 (37.1–43.5)	49.8 (46.1–53.4)	50.1 (46.1–54.0)	38.7 (35.6–41.9)	42.0 (38.8–45.1)	26.6 (23.0–30.2)	32.1 (28.4–35.9)
Knowledge	23.7 (22.4–25.1)	23.2 (21.8–24.5)	18.9 (16.1–21.7)	19.7 (17.1–22.3)	25.7 (22.6–28.7)	19.0 (15.7–22.4)	26.0 (23.2–28.8)	26.3 (23.4–29.1)	24.9 (21.5–28.3)	23.2 (19.6–26.7)
Attitudes	73.2 (71.8–74.6)	75.9 (74.5–77.3)	75.7 (72.7–78.6)	77.7 (74.9–80.5)	66.1 (62.6–69.6)	66.7 (62.9–70.5)	70.1 (67.2–73.1)	73.0 (70.0–76.0)	72.7 (69.3–76.1)	78.6 (75.0–82.2)
Liking	69.6 (68.2–71.1)	74.3 (72.8–75.7)	70.9 (67.8–74.0)	77.4 (74.5–80.3)	71.2 (67.8–74.5)	72.8 (69.2–76.5)	72.3 (69.4–75.2)	74.0 (71.1–77.0)	76.3 (73.0–79.5)	82.9 (79.6–86.3)
General self-efficacy	71.1 (69.7–72.5)	76.0 (74.6–77.4)	70.6 (67.5–73.7)	75.0 (72.1–78.0)	72.9 (69.7–76.0)	79.9 (76.5–83.3)	75.6 (72.8–78.4)	76.2 (73.4–79.0)	73.8 (70.6–77.0)	84.9 (81.5–88.3)
Intention	50.5 (48.9–52.1)	57.4 (55.9–59.0)	48.9 (45.3–52.4)	56.3 (52.9–59.6)	43.8 (40.2–47.5)	49.4 (45.5–53.4)	55.4 (52.2–58.6)	64.1 (61.0–67.3)	63.4 (59.7–67.1)	72.7 (68.8–76.6)
Habit	40.8 (39.2–42.4)	46.6 (45.0–48.2)	38.0 (34.4–41.5)	45.6 (42.2–48.9)	45.2 (41.6–48.9)	50.8 (46.9–54.8)	40.2 (37.0–43.4)	44.1 (40.9–47.3)	38.5 (34.6–42.4)	45.0 (40.9–49.1)
Preferences	60.6 (59.0–62.1)	62.1 (60.5–63.7)	66.9 (63.7–70.1)	71.8 (68.7–74.9)	73.0 (69.8–76.2)	75.7 (72.2–79.1)	56.5 (53.3–59.8)	56.7 (53.4–59.9)	65.7 (61.9–69.5)	67.3 (63.3–71.3)
Perceived barriers	22.4 (21.1–23.6)	15.3 (14.0–16.5)	32.2 (29.2–35.2)	19.0 (16.2–21.9)	23.0 (20.1–25.9)	15.8 (12.7–19.0)	20.5 (18.2–22.9)	12.0 (9.6–14.4)	16.9 (14.2–19.5)	8.0 (5.3–10.7)
Perceived social environment										
Subjective norm/ modelling	58.9 (57.4–60.5)	62.9 (61.3–64.4)	64.1 (60.8–67.5)	64.8 (61.6–67.9)	60.8 (57.3–64.4)	64.4 (60.6–68.3)	49.7 (46.5–52.9)	51.3 (48.1–54.6)	44.9 (40.9–48.8)	52.3 (48.1–56.4)
Active parental encouragement	50.2 (48.6–51.8)	54.1 (52.5–55.7)	46.5 (43.0–50.0)	50.1 (46.8–53.5)	54.9 (51.3–58.5)	54.8 (50.8–58.7)	36.1 (33.0–39.2)	36.4 (33.3–39.5)	47.5 (43.5–51.4)	50.5 (46.4–54.7)
Demand family rule	39.8 (38.2–41.4)	43.8 (42.2–45.3)	25.8 (22.7–28.9)	26.4 (23.4–29.3)	38.8 (35.2–42.4)	42.6 (38.7–46.4)	33.7 (30.7–36.7)	31.5 (28.5–34.6)	32.6 (28.7–36.4)	38.3 (34.3–42.2)
Allow family rule	79.5 (78.2–80.7)	83.5 (82.2–84.7)	89.7 (87.6–91.7)	91.5 (89.6–93.5)	75.4 (72.3–78.5)	79.0 (75.6–82.3)	81.7 (79.3–84.1)	85.2 (82.7–87.6)	81.0 (78.1–83.9)	88.4 (85.4–91.4)
Parental facilitation	24.8 (23.4–26.1)	24.4 (23.0–25.8)	30.5 (27.2–33.8)	29.3 (26.2–32.4)	11.5 (9.3–13.7)	8.7 (6.3–11.1)	19.4 (16.9–22.0)	18.8 (16.2–21.4)	20.4 (17.2–23.5)	17.6 (14.3–20.8)
Perceived physical environment										
Availability at home	73.5 (72.2–74.9)	77.8 (76.4–79.1)	76.4 (73.6–79.3)	81.1 (78.4–83.8)	66.7 (63.3–70.1)	69.8 (66.1–73.5)	75.8 (73.0–78.5)	76.7 (73.9–79.5)	62.9 (59.1–66.6)	68.5 (64.5–72.4)
Availability at school and leisure	13.9 (12.8–15.0)	13.8 (12.7–14.9)	21.3 (18.3–24.2)	22.8 (20.0–25.6)	14.1 (11.5–16.7)	14.4 (11.7–17.2)	19.2 (16.6–21.8)	18.4 (15.8–21.1)	5.7 (3.9–7.5)	4.9 (3.1–6.8)

variations (ranging from a low of about 10% in Belgium and the Netherlands to a high of 51% in Portugal). No substantial gender differences were seen for this item. However, a consistently larger proportion of girls reported positively on the other social factors than did boys. The north-south gradient found in social-environmental factors for fruit could not be detected for vegetables. However, fewer children in the Nordic countries (with the exception of Sweden) and in Spain reported positively on modelling compared to children in Sweden, Portugal and the Netherlands. About one third of the children in Denmark and of boys in Norway reported positively on parental encouragement compared to around 70% of the Portuguese children. Few Norwegian (20%) and Austrian children (25%) said their parents demanded that they eat vegetables every day compared to about 65% for the Dutch and Portuguese children.

Environmental Factors

Overall, about 75% of the children reported that vegetables were available at their home always or on most days. In contrast, only 14% reported that vegetables were available at school, at their friends' house or at other places for leisure time activities. More than half the children said they can never get vegetables at school, while 20% said they can never get vegetables at their friends' house when spending the afternoon there. The corresponding figure for leisure time activity arenas was 43% (results not shown in table 3). Country differences in availability at school and during leisure time activities were also large, as only 1–2% of the Dutch children, about 6% of Icelandic and Spanish children, around 20% of Danish and Austrian children and as many as 30% of the Swedish children reported that vegetables were available at school and places for leisure time activities most days or always.

Table 3 (continued)

Constructs	Countries									
	Netherlands		Norway		Portugal		Spain		Sweden	
	M	F	M	F	M	F	M	F	M	F
Personal										
Self-rated intake	52.6 (48.2–57.0)	54.4 (50.4–58.4)	35.9 (31.9–40.0)	45.7 (41.7–49.8)	31.4 (28.5–34.3)	31.8 (29.1–34.5)	28.7 (25.2–32.1)	34.3 (30.5–38.0)	37.5 (33.8–41.1)	41.9 (38.2–45.5)
Knowledge	23.9 (20.3–27.6)	20.5 (17.2–23.9)	19.7 (16.5–23.0)	18.7 (15.5–22.0)	37.6 (34.6–40.7)	38.6 (35.8–41.5)	12.9 (10.5–15.3)	10.8 (8.2–13.4)	17.3 (14.4–20.2)	18.6 (15.7–21.5)
Attitudes	68.9 (64.8–73.0)	69.6 (65.8–73.4)	74.8 (71.3–78.3)	79.8 (76.2–83.3)	81.8 (79.4–84.1)	84.5 (82.3–86.7)	71.1 (67.7–74.6)	72.8 (69.1–76.5)	73.2 (69.9–76.5)	74.5 (71.2–77.9)
Liking	68.7 (64.8–72.7)	76.2 (72.5–79.8)	74.2 (70.9–77.6)	84.8 (81.5–88.1)	67.4 (64.5–70.3)	69.4 (66.6–72.1)	53.5 (49.6–57.4)	53.2 (49.0–57.4)	72.1 (68.8–75.3)	79.7 (76.5–83.0)
General self-efficacy	78.0 (74.4–81.6)	79.5 (76.2–82.8)	76.4 (73.1–79.7)	84.0 (80.7–87.3)	64.6 (61.7–67.5)	69.7 (67.0–72.5)	54.3 (50.6–58.1)	57.3 (53.2–61.3)	78.3 (75.3–81.3)	82.7 (79.7–85.7)
Intention	49.8 (45.4–54.1)	58.8 (54.8–62.9)	57.3 (53.3–61.2)	70.9 (67.0–74.8)	52.4 (49.3–55.5)	52.3 (49.3–55.2)	31.9 (28.4–35.4)	34.5 (30.7–38.3)	51.7 (48.0–55.4)	61.0 (57.3–64.7)
Habit	56.5 (52.2–60.7)	65.8 (61.9–69.7)	39.2 (35.0–43.3)	49.3 (45.2–53.4)	44.5 (41.4–47.6)	47.2 (44.3–50.1)	30.5 (27.0–33.9)	29.3 (25.6–33.0)	38.0 (34.3–41.7)	43.5 (39.8–47.2)
Preferences	65.0 (60.8–69.1)	69.7 (66.0–73.5)	59.3 (55.2–63.4)	61.5 (57.5–65.5)	62.2 (59.1–65.2)	62.1 (59.2–64.9)	44.1 (40.3–47.9)	45.3 (41.3–49.3)	52.2 (48.4–56.0)	49.4 (45.6–53.2)
Perceived barriers	14.1 (11.3–16.9)	9.0 (6.4–11.5)	16.6 (13.7–19.6)	12.4 (9.5–15.3)	25.2 (22.6–27.7)	20.2 (17.7–22.6)	34.1 (30.6–37.6)	28.4 (24.7–32.1)	12.3 (10.0–14.6)	9.3 (6.9–11.6)
Perceived social environment										
Subjective norm/ modelling	72.6 (68.9–76.4)	78.7 (75.3–82.2)	50.6 (46.5–54.8)	53.7 (49.6–57.9)	68.9 (66.0–71.8)	68.1 (65.4–70.9)	48.9 (45.1–52.7)	56.2 (52.2–60.3)	69.1 (65.6–72.5)	73.7 (70.3–77.1)
Active parental encouragement	56.4 (52.1–60.8)	59.4 (55.4–63.4)	36.2 (32.1–40.2)	44.4 (40.4–48.5)	66.9 (64.0–69.8)	71.2 (68.5–73.9)	56.8 (53.0–60.5)	61.8 (57.8–65.7)	48.1 (44.4–51.9)	53.6 (49.8–57.3)
Demand family rule	60.6 (56.5–64.7)	71.7 (67.9–75.5)	20.8 (17.4–24.2)	22.0 (18.7–25.4)	64.3 (61.3–67.3)	64.7 (61.9–67.6)	45.2 (41.4–49.0)	48.8 (44.8–52.9)	33.8 (30.2–37.4)	41.1 (37.5–44.7)
Allow family rule	79.2 (75.7–82.6)	83.1 (79.9–86.3)	74.7 (71.4–78.0)	85.0 (81.8–88.3)	75.4 (72.7–78.1)	76.1 (73.6–78.6)	69.4 (65.9–72.8)	73.6 (69.9–77.3)	86.7 (84.3–89.0)	91.2 (88.8–93.5)
Parental facilitation	9.4 (6.7–12.0)	10.7 (8.3–13.2)	17.2 (14.1–20.3)	16.0 (12.9–19.0)	51.0 (47.9–54.1)	51.0 (48.1–54.0)	16.3 (13.5–19.0)	15.5 (12.6–18.5)	31.1 (27.6–34.5)	28.8 (25.4–32.2)
Perceived physical environment										
Availability at home	72.0 (68.2–75.9)	75.4 (71.9–79.0)	66.9 (63.1–70.7)	74.5 (70.7–78.2)	81.0 (78.5–83.4)	81.6 (79.3–83.9)	73.4 (70.3–76.6)	81.0 (77.6–84.4)	79.6 (76.8–82.5)	85.5 (82.7–88.3)
Availability at school and leisure	2.3 (1.1–3.5)	1.6 (0.5–2.8)	8.1 (5.8–10.4)	7.8 (5.6–10.1)	12.3 (10.3–14.4)	12.2 (10.2–14.1)	7.2 (5.4–9.0)	5.0 (3.0–6.9)	27.9 (24.5–31.4)	30.2 (26.7–33.6)

Discussion

Results from this study indicate that European children hold positive attitudes towards fruit and vegetable consumption. Overall, they are more positive towards fruit than towards vegetables. Knowledge of what constitutes an adequate intake of fruit and vegetable seems to be rather low as only slightly more than half of the children knew the fruit guidelines and fewer than 1 in 4 children knew the vegetable guidelines. It may be that children at this age have difficulties in distinguishing between fruit and vegetables. Also, the current recommendations differ between different countries [1], which complicates the procedure of ascertaining these children's exact level of knowledge.

In general, the children report that they experience the social environment as supportive towards fruit and vegetable intake. For social factors regarding fruit, we found a clear north-south difference in parental modelling, demand and active encouragement, but this could not be detected for vegetables. It may be that this pattern is reflecting the more traditional north-south gradient in fruit and vegetable consumption among adults shown in several studies [16, 17], and that as food cultures are changing and may be subject to 'globalization', this gradient is gradually disappearing. Fruit is more or less ready to eat, whereas vegetables more often demand cooking and preparation. It may be that the social factors regarding fruit consumption are more robust against cultural changes than the ones regarding vegetable intake.

We also found a large difference in parental facilitation across countries, both for fruit and for vegetables. One could argue that the different proportions of parents cutting fruit/vegetables for their children in the different countries reflect differing views in what children at this age can do for themselves and what they need help with. Another possibility is that parents in some countries believe they should encourage health behaviour more actively in these young adolescents, compared to other countries. However, it has been shown that cutting up fruit or vegetables increases intake for children as such, by making eating it easier [18]. In this paper, parents cutting up fruit and vegetables for their children has been defined as a social-environmental factor since it could be seen as an act of direct social support. However, cutting up fruit and vegetables may also improve accessibility of these items at home. It may be that even though children perceive fruit and vegetables to be highly available at home, increasing accessibility may also be necessary in order to increase their consumption, in particular among children with low preferences [19]. Further analysis will clarify the relationship between these factors and fruit and vegetable intake.

The children reported a high availability of fruit and vegetables at home, but perceived fruit and vegetable availability outside home as low, particularly at school and at leisure time activities. Also, large differences between countries were detected both for fruit and for vegetable availability outside home. This may reflect differences in fruit and vegetable subscription, lunch schemes and other buying possibilities at school in the different countries. For example, the higher perceived availability of vegetables at school and leisure time in Sweden probably reflects the vegetables in the daily, warm school meal served in Swedish schools. Further analysis of the data is warranted to relate country differences in these availability factors with information collected on food availability and food school policies in the Pro Children countries.

For personal factors regarding vegetable intake, we found that the Spanish children were substantially less positive than the other children. Intake data also showed that Spanish children consume fewer vegetables than most of the other children in the Pro Children study, with the exception of the Icelandic children [1]. Further analysis is needed, within countries as well as between countries, to see whether the rather surprising differences in liking, self-efficacy, intention and perceived barriers are correlated with differences in observed intakes.

We did not find a clear and consistent pattern for between-country differences for other factors than aforementioned. There was, however, a large variation between countries both in personal, social and environmental factors. A clear-cut north-south dimension was only detected for social factors related to fruit, and none of the other potential determinants. More in-depth analysis of data for each country, as well as multilevel analysis for the full survey population is necessary in order to explore which factors are more important for which children in the different countries.

For fruit as well as for vegetables, somewhat higher scores were found for girls than for boys on the personal, social and environmental factors. However, substantial differences between genders within each country were mostly found in the Nordic countries, and why this is the case needs further investigation, perhaps leading to gender-tailored intervention tools.

The Pro Children study applies a standardized, validated instrument to measure fruit and vegetable intake and its potential psychosocial correlates across diverse food-related cultural settings. However, the questionnaire contained more than 100 items and clearly was a demanding instrument to respond to for young children. Some children were unable to complete the questionnaire during a school lesson of 45 min. However, the test-retest reliability was either good or very good for 24 out of 30 constructs, and acceptable for the remaining [12], which indicates that children at this age were able to respond to the instrument in a meaningful manner.

Internal consistency measured by Cronbach's α was good or acceptable for all scales, except for the self-efficacy scale for fruit and for vegetables. Martens et al. [20] measured self-efficacy in a similar manner for adolescents in the Netherlands and reported an even lower inter-item correlation of 0.34 for self-efficacy regarding fruit intake. Evidently, low reliability of a measure of a potential determinant may obscure relations between this factor and intake [19], which should be avoided, and the reliability of the self-efficacy measure should be improved before the Pro Children questionnaire is being used in future studies. Furthermore, in further analyses of the Pro Children data set, the low reliability of the self-efficacy scales should be kept in mind when interpreting the findings from these analyses.

By dichotomising the scales as done in this paper, one looses variation in the constructs. However, running the analysis presented in tables 2 and 3 on the full scales (with mean scores and standard deviations) revealed a pattern similar to the one presented. Thus, we chose to report and discuss proportions and confidence intervals in order to increase the readability and ease of interpretation of the data presented. Future analyses will present more detailed descriptions of and associations between the constructs presented in the present paper.

In the result part, we chose to report confidence intervals instead of p values, and to comment on results in terms of differences that were not only statistically significant but also believed to be of practical importance. Because of the large sample size, almost all gender differences for the full sample are statistically significant. Furthermore, application of a strict Bonferroni correction based on the large number tests to study within- and between-country differences increased the risk of making type 2 errors. Nevertheless, all gender differences commented on for the full sample were significant at a 0.001 level, whereas all gender differences within countries were significant at least at a 0.02 level.

All data reported in this paper are based on self-reports, with its inherent limitations (for a critique, see Young et al. [21]). However, it is the only way to assess the beliefs, feelings and experiences of people [11], and when we are aiming at capturing perceptions, attitudes and beliefs, these limitations do not necessarily cause problems. Self-report data may still create a threat to the validity of this study by the possible existence of a pleasing effect, creating artificially high values on the psychosocial factors. However, the study was carried out anonymously, and reported intake of fruit and vegetables was low [1], which may be evidence against the interplay of such an effect. Still, the gender differences detected in this study could be the result of a pleasing effect, since girls might be more eager to please than boys. However, for constructs like availability outside home, as well as for parental facilitation, no gender differences or small differences in the opposite direction were detected, which speaks against the existence of a general pleasing effect affecting girls' replies only.

The questionnaire was developed with the aim to be fully comparative between countries [6]. Therefore, all language versions contained the same items, in the same order. Every effort was made to avoid differences in meaning and interpretation of words and phrases. Procedures of data collection were standardized as much as possible to minimize the effect this may have on the results. Still, we cannot rule out that cultural differences in how items and questions were interpreted, and that between-country differences in children's ability to accurately self-report based on skills, prior experience and interpretation may have affected the results. However, test-retest reliability scores were quite similar across the 5 participating countries in the test-retest sample, indicating that this was not a major problem in this study [12].

There are three possible levels of attrition in this study: individuals, classes and schools. Individuals because they or their parents did not want to participate, or because the children were absent for other reasons the day the questionnaires were completed. Classes and schools because teachers and/or headmasters did not want to participate. There is reason to believe that the latter did not cause systematic attrition – there are probably no characteristics or qualities of the individual students that affected the teacher's or headmaster's decision not to participate. For the individual level, almost all children present at the day the study was carried out participated, and only 144 out of nearly 14,000 questionnaires were destroyed on parents' request. This probably did not affect the results to a large degree. Thus, the trends, differences and country variation described above probably reflect real differences between these countries.

The Pro Children study applied a standardized, validated instrument to measure fruit and vegetable intake and its potential psychosocial and environmental correlates in relatively large representative samples in nine European countries with a high participation rate. Results showed that in general, children in the countries studied have a positive attitude towards fruit and vegetable consumption; they like fruit and vegetables and have a high preference for fruit. Despite this, their fruit and vegetable intakes are well below recommended levels for all countries [1]. Thus, there is a strong need for interventions that should include attempts to improve availability and accessibility of fruit and vegetables outside the home environment, particularly at school. Further analytical studies are needed to quantify the relationship between these factors and intake to see whether the personal, social and environmental factors described in the present study are indeed associated with and predict fruit and vegetable intakes.

Acknowledgements

This study is being carried out with financial support from the Commission of the European Communities, specific RTD programme 'Quality of Life and Management of Living Resources', QLK1-2001-00547 'Promoting and Sustaining Health through Increased Fruit and Vegetable Consumption among European Schoolchildren' (Pro Children). The study does not necessarily reflect the Commission's views and in no way anticipates the Commission's future policy in this area. The authors want to thank all children who participated in the Pro Children survey; all school staff, headmasters and teachers who kindly accepted to be involved in the study, and finally all project staff and students from all nine participating countries who coordinated the survey and entered the data.

Appendix: Internal consistency for constructs related to fruit/vegetable intake

Construct with item(s)	Response categories	Internal consistency Cronbach's α	
		Fruit	Vegetables
Personal			
Self-rated intake			
Do you think that you eat much or a little fruit/many or few vegetables? Do you think that you eat more or less fruit/vegetables than most boys and girls of your age?	5-point scale from 1 = very much to 5 = very little 1 = much more to 5 = much less	0.74	0.77
Knowledge			
How much fruit do you think you should eat to have a healthy diet?	1 = no fruit, 2 = 1–3 pieces per week, 3 = 4–6 pieces per week, 4 = 1 piece per day, 5 = 2 pieces per day, 6 = 3 pieces per day, 7 = 4 pieces per day, 8 = 5 pieces per day or more	–	
How many vegetables do you think you should eat to have a healthy diet?	1 = no vegetables, 2 = 1–3 portions (serving spoons) per week, 3 = 4–6 portions per week, 4 = 1 portion every day, 5 = 2 portions every day, 6 = 3 portions every day, 7 = 4 portions every day, 8 = 5 or more portions every day		–
Attitudes			
To eat fruit/vegetables every day makes me feel good To eat fruit/vegetables every day gives me more energy	5-point scale from 1 = I fully agree to 5 = I fully disagree	0.73	0.84
Liking			
I like to eat fruit/vegetables every day Fruit tastes good/vegetables taste good	5-point scale from 1 = I fully agree to 5 = I fully disagree	0.68	0.84
General self-efficacy			
It is difficult for me to eat fruit/vegetables every day[1] If I decide to eat fruit/vegetables every day, I can do it	5-point scale from 1 = I fully agree to 5 = I fully disagree	0.39	0.43
Intention			
I want to eat fruit/vegetables every day	5-point scale from 1 = I fully agree to 5 = I fully disagree	–	–
Habit			
To eat fruit/vegetables every day is a habit for me	5-point scale from 1 = I fully agree to 5 = I fully disagree	–	–
Preferences fruit			
Which of the following fruits do you like or dislike? List of 12 fruits: apple, bananas, pears, oranges, tangerines, plums, peaches, melon, strawberries, grapes, cherries, kiwis	4-point scale from 1 = like very much to 4 = dislike very much and 5 = have not tried	–	–

Construct with item(s)	Response categories	Internal consistency Cronbach's α	
		Fruit	Vegetables
Preferences vegetables			
Which of the following vegetables do you like or dislike? List of 12 vegetables: tomatoes, cucumber, salad, cabbage, spinach, leak, green beans, onion, carrots, broccoli, cauliflower, green peas	4-point scale from 1 = like very much to 4 = dislike very much and 5 = have not tried	–	–
Perceived barriers fruit			
I do not eat fruit because it takes too much time to eat I do not eat fruit because I want to eat something else (e.g. sweets) I do not eat fruit because my fingers get greasy when I eat it I do not eat fruit because it gets squeezed in the schoolbag	5-point scale from 1 = I fully agree to 5 = I fully disagree	0.72	–
Perceived barriers vegetables			
I do not eat vegetables because it takes too much time to eat I do not eat vegetables because I am still hungry after having eaten them I do not eat vegetables because I want to eat something else (e.g. sweets) I do not eat vegetables because they get squeezed in the schoolbag	5-point scale from 1 = I fully agree to 5 = I fully disagree	–	0.79
Perceived social environmental			
Subjective norm/modelling			
My mother eats fruit/vegetables every day My father eats fruit/vegetables every day My best friends eat fruit/vegetables every day	5-point scale from 1 = I fully agree to 5 = I fully disagree and 6 = I don't have/don't see my mother/father	0.59	0.71
Active parental encouragement			
My mother encourages me to eat fruit/vegetables every day My father encourages me to eat fruit/vegetables every day	5-point scale from 1 = I fully agree to 5 = I fully disagree and 6 = I don't have/don't see my mother/father	0.82	0.88
Demand family rule			
Do your parents demand that you eat fruit/vegetables every day?	5-point scale from 1 = yes, always to 5 = never	–	–
Allow family rule			
Are you allowed to eat as much fruit/as many vegetables as you like at home?	5-point scale from 1 = yes, always to 5 = never	–	–
Parental facilitation			
Does your mother or father usually cut up fruit/vegetables for you in between meals?	5-point scale from 1 = yes, always to 5 = never	–	–
Perceived physical environmental			
Availability at home			
If you tell at home what fruit/which vegetables you would like to eat, will it be bought? Are there usually different kinds of fruits/vegetables available in your home? Is/are there usually fruit/vegetables available at home that you like?	5-point scale from 1 = yes, always to 5 = never	0.54	0.68
Availability at school and leisure			
Can you get fruit/vegetable at school either by buying it or getting it for free? Can you get fruit/vegetables at your friends' house, when you spend the afternoon there? Can you get fruit/vegetable at the place where you have your leisure time activity (e.g. club, sports place), either by buying it or getting it for free?	5-point scale from 1 = yes, always to 5 = never	0.43	0.54

[1] This item is recoded before the scale is computed, so that all items are coded in the same direction.

References

1 Yngve A, Wolf A, Poortvliet E, Elmadfa I, Brug J, Ehrenblad B, Franchini B, Haraldsdóttir J, Krølner R, Maes L, Pérez-Rodrigo C, Sjöström M, Thórsdóttir I, Klepp K-I: Fruit and vegetable intake in a sample of 11-year-old children in 9 European countries: the Pro Children cross-sectional survey. Ann Nutr Metab 2005;49:236–245.

2 Kelder SH, Perry CL, Klepp K-I, Lytle L: Longitudinal tracking of adolescent smoking, physical activity and food choice behaviors. Am J Public Health 1994;84:1121–1126.

3 Lien N, Lytle LA, Klepp K-I: Stability in consumption of fruit, vegetables, and sugary foods in a cohort from age 14 to 21. Prev Med 2001; 33:217–226.

4 Mikkilä V, Räsänen L, Raitakari OT, Pietinen P, Viikari J: Longitudinal changes in diet from childhood into adulthood with respect to risk of cardiovascular diseases: the Cardiovascular Risk in Young Finns Study. Eur J Clin Nutr 2004;58:1038–1045.

5 Bartholomew LK, Parcel, GS, Kok G, Gottlieb N: Intervention Mapping: A Process for Designing Theory- and Evidence-Based Health Education Programs. Mountain View, Mayfield, 2001.

6 Klepp K-I, Pérez-Rodrigo C, De Bourdeaudhuij I, Due P, Elmadfa I, Haraldsdóttir J, König J, Sjöström M, Thórsdóttir I, de Almeida MDV, Yngve A, Brug J: Promoting fruit and vegetable consumption among European schoolchildren: rationale, conceptualization and design of the Pro Children Project. Ann Nutr Metab 2005;49:212–220.

7 Domel SB, Thompson WO, Davis HC, Baranowski T, Leonard SB, Baranowski J: Psychosocial predictors of fruit and vegetable consumption among elementary school children. Health Educ Res 1996;11:299–308.

8 Resnicow K, Davis-Hearn M, Smith M, Baranowski T, Lin LS, Baranowski J, Doyle C, Wang DT: Social-cognitive predictors of fruit and vegetable intake in children. Health Psychol 1997;16:272–276.

9 Reynolds KD, Hinton AW, Shewchuk RM, Hickey CA: Social cognitive model of fruit and vegetable consumption in elementary school children. J Nutr Educ 1999;31:23–30.

10 Neumark-Sztainer D, Wall M, Perry C, Story M: Correlates of fruit and vegetable intake among adolescents. Findings from Project EAT. Prev Med 2003;37:198–208.

11 Baranowski T, Cullen KW, Baranowski J: Psychosocial correlates of dietary intake: advancing dietary intervention. Ann Rev Nutr 1999; 19:17–40.

12 De Bourdeaudhuij I, Klepp K-I, Due P, Pérez-Rodrigo C, de Almeida MDV, Wind M, Krølner R, Sandvik C, Brug J: Reliability and validity of a questionnaire to measure personal, social and environmental correlates of fruit and vegetable intake in 10- to 11-year-old children in five European countries. Public Health Nutr 2005;8:189–200.

13 Baranowski T, Lin LS, Wetter DW, Resnicow K, Hearn MD: Theory as mediating variables: why aren't community interventions working as desired? Ann Epidemiol 1997;S7:S89–S95.

14 Gibson EL, Wardle J, Watts CJ: Fruit and vegetable consumption, nutritional knowledge and beliefs in mothers and children. Appetite 1998;31:205–228.

15 Bere E: Increasing Schoolchildren's Intake of Fruit and Vegetables. Fruits and Vegetables Make the Marks; thesis, Oslo, 2003.

16 Elmadfa I, Weichselbaum E, Koenig J, Remaut De Winter A-M, Trolle E, Haapala I, et al: European nutrition and health report 2004. Executive Summary. Ann Nutr Metab 2004; 48(suppl 2):1–16.

17 Agudo A, Slimani N, Ocke MC, Naska A, Miller AB, Kroke A, et al: Consumption of vegetables, fruit and other plant foods in the European Prospective Investigation into Cancer and Nutrition (EPIC) cohorts from 10 European countries. Public Health Nutr 2002;5: 1179–1196.

18 Bönnhoff N, Eissing G, Baumann T, Kuss S: Steigerung des Obst- und Gemüseverzehrs bei Grundschulkindern. Ernährungs-Umschau 2002;49:340–343.

19 Cullen KW, Baranowski T, Owens E, Marsh T, Rittenberry L, de Moor C: Availability, accessibility and preferences for fruit, 100% fruit juice and vegetables influence children's dietary behavior. Health Educ Behav 2003;30: 645–626.

20 Martens MK, van Assema P, Brug J: Why do adolescents eat what they eat? Personal and social environmental predictors of fruit, snack and breakfast consumption among Dutch 12- to 14-year-old students. Public Health Nutr 2005; in press.

21 Young EM, Fors SW, Hayes DM: Associations between perceived parent behaviors and middle school student fruit and vegetable consumption. J Nutr Educ Behav 2004;36:2–12.

Annals of
Nutrition&
Metabolism

Ann Nutr Metab 2005;49:267–277
DOI: 10.1159/000087249

Published online: July 28, 2005

The Pro Children Intervention: Applying the Intervention Mapping Protocol to Develop a School-Based Fruit and Vegetable Promotion Programme

Carmen Pérez-Rodrigo[a] Marianne Wind[b] Christina Hildonen[c]
Mona Bjelland[c] Javier Aranceta[a] Knut-Inge Klepp[c] Johannes Brug[b]

[a]Community Nutrition Unit, Department of Public Health, Bilbao, Spain; [b]Department of Public Health, Erasmus University Medical Center Rotterdam, Rotterdam, The Netherlands; [c]Department of Nutrition, Faculty of Medicine, University of Oslo, Oslo, Norway

Key Words
Intervention mapping · Determinants of fruit and vegetable intake · Food habits · School setting

Abstract
Background/Aims: The importance of careful theory-based intervention planning is recognized for fruit and vegetable promotion. This paper describes the application of the Intervention Mapping (IM) protocol to develop the Pro Children intervention to promote consumption of fruit and vegetable among 10- to 13-year-old schoolchildren. ***Methods:*** Based on a needs assessment, promotion of intake of fruit and vegetable was split into performance objectives and related personal, social and environmental determinants. Crossing the performance objectives with related important and changeable determinants resulted in a matrix of learning and change objectives for which appropriate educational strategies were identified. Theoretically similar but culturally relevant interventions were designed, implemented and evaluated in Norway, the Netherlands and Spain during 2 school years. ***Results:*** Programme activities included provision of fruits and vegetables in the schools, guided classroom activities, computer-tailored feedback and advice for children, and activities to be completed at home with the family. Additionally, optional intervention components for community reinforcement included incorporation of mass media, school health services or grocery stores. School project committees were supported. ***Conclusion:*** The Pro Children intervention was carefully developed based on the IM protocol that resulted in a comprehensive school-based fruit and vegetable promotion programme, but culturally sensible and locally relevant.

Introduction

As shown by available evidence, fruit and vegetable intake is too low among European schoolchildren [1, 2]. School-based health promotion strategies fostering healthy eating practices have the potential to improve health and well-being during childhood and later stages in life [3, 4]. The Pro Children consortium aimed to initiate, develop, implement and evaluate school-based fruit and vegetable promotion actions among primary school-

KARGER
Fax +41 61 306 12 34
E-Mail karger@karger.ch
www.karger.com

0250–6807/05/0494–0267$22.00/0

Accessible online at:
www.karger.com/anm

Carmen Pérez-Rodrigo
Department of Public Health, Community Nutrition Unit
Luis Briñas, 18; 4th floor
ES–48013 Bilbao (Spain)
Tel. +34 94 4204465, Fax +34 94 4204466, E-Mail bisaludpublica@wanadoo.es

children aged 10–13 years in different European countries [4]. This consortium especially aimed to develop an evidence-based and theory-driven intervention package that is applicable in different European countries.

Since the publication of the Precede-Proceed model by Green and Kreuter [5] and other similar health promotion planning models [6], the importance of careful theory-based intervention planning is recognized. According to such planning models (fig. 1), the first phase (A) in health promotion planning is the identification of health problems that are serious and/or prevalent. In the second phase (B), the behavioural risk factors for the health problems need to be identified. Phase C is to investigate the individual and environmental mediators or determinants of these risk behaviours. These determinants should then be translated into interventions (phase D) that can be implemented and disseminated (phase E).

Within the aforementioned planning models, the road map to *what* needs to be changed is well laid out. Phases A–C lead to evidence-based indications about which health problems need to be addressed, which health behaviours need to be changed, as well as which behavioural determinants need to be influenced. Health promotion planning models thus give good guidance on selecting specific change objectives, but are less specific in *how* change should be induced, i.e. how the objectives should be translated into effective interventions. Intervention Mapping (IM) [7–9] was especially developed for this purpose. Furthermore, IM recognizes the importance of social ecological models of behaviour change, thus highlighting individual motivational factors as well as environmental opportunities as important mediators of health behaviour. Earlier studies show that dietary habits of children may be largely dependent on such environmental factors [10]. IM was therefore selected as the framework to develop fruit and vegetable promotion interventions for schoolchildren.

In this paper, we will first introduce the IM protocol and subsequently describe how we applied the IM protocol to the development of the Pro Children intervention.

Intervention Mapping

IM is a stepwise approach to ensure a systematic evidence-based and theory-driven development and implementation of health promotion interventions. IM structures the initiation, development and implementation of such interventions based on established theories and empirical data. IM guides the selection of specified intervention goals, the choice of intervention strategies and the development of intervention tools. It also prepares the adoption, implementation and evaluation of the intervention. IM is thus a specification of phases D and E of the planning model depicted in figure 1. It assumes that phases A–C have been carefully conducted and refers to these phases as the 'needs assessment'. To complete this needs assessment, IM proposes to use a combination of qualitative and quantitative research methods, starting with reviewing the literature on relevant evidence and theories. Since the body of evidence on health and behaviour is in general much stronger than for behavioural determinants, it is often especially necessary to conduct additional research to further explore the determinants of target behaviours [9, 11]. IM proposes to use social ecological models that recognize the importance of individual, social and environmental factors as important determinants of health behaviours.

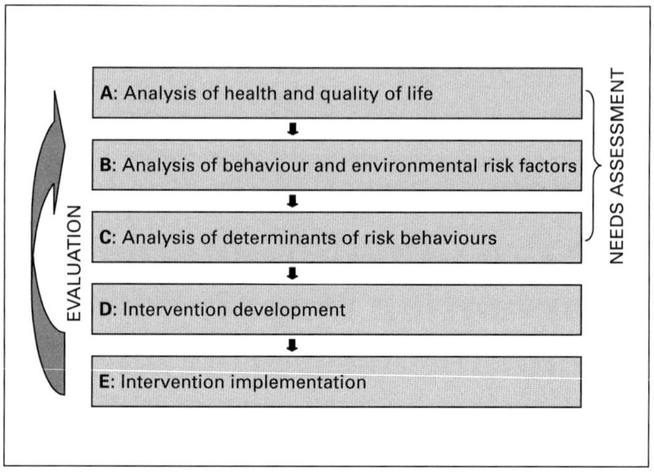

Fig. 1. A simple model for planned health education and promotion.

IM then recognizes 5 steps, from the definition of specific intervention objectives to the development of an evaluation plan (fig. 2). IM assumes a temporal order from step 1 to step 5, but certainly allows and encourages a more iterative process, i.e. going back to an earlier step if this seems necessary.

At step 1 of IM, proximal programme goals are specified based on the needs assessment. These goals are referred to as performance objectives: the specific behaviours people in the target group need to participate in, or the specific changes to be achieved in the environment as

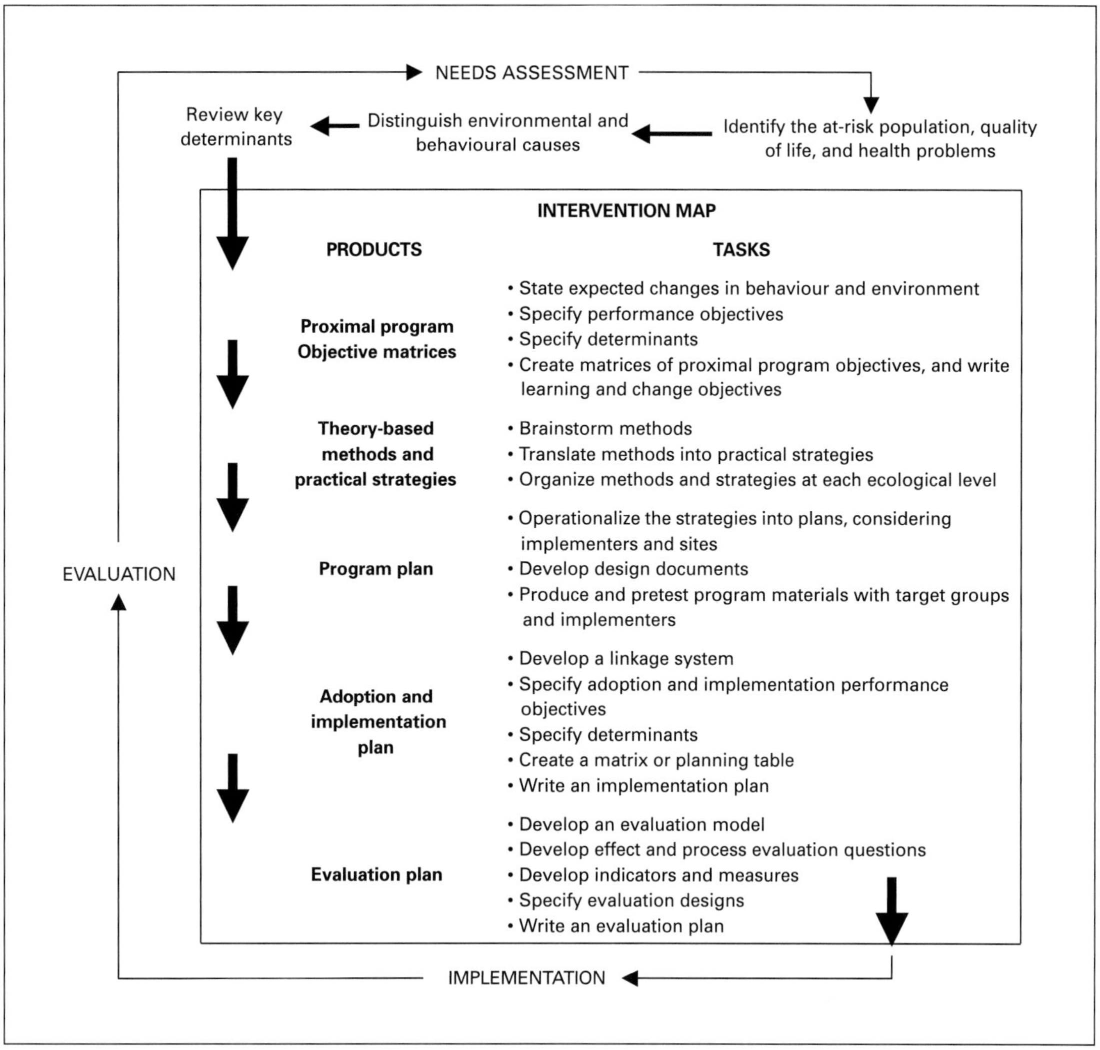

Fig. 2. Protocol for the IM planning procedure. Source: Bartholomew et al. [7].

a result of the programme. Important and changeable determinants of these performance objectives should be selected. Combinations of selected determinants and performance objectives are then used to specify the most proximal learning and environmental change objectives. Matrices are constructed to facilitate that process. For personal determinants, learning objectives intend to answer the question 'What does the target group need to learn with regard to a specific determinant in order to accomplish the performance objective?' In the same way, considering determinants at the family and school level, change objectives need to answer: 'What needs to change in the environment to enable the target group to reach the performance objective?'

At step 2, a list of theory-based and evidence-based intervention methods is generated that matches the learning objectives. Subsequently these theoretical methods are translated into practical intervention strategies. Step 3 is the design of the actual programme. This requires organizing the strategies into a deliverable programme, considering the target groups and the settings. Furthermore, the actual educational materials have to be selected, produced and pretested. At step 4, the plan for the implementation of the programme is developed which should highlight the anticipated prerequisites for successful programme adoption and dissemination. Adoption and diffusion of an intervention programme is, of course, crucial for its success and it often requires tailoring the

Table 1. Identified changeable important determinants of fruit and vegetable consumption in the Pro Children intervention

Personal determinants	Social determinants	Environmental determinants
Awareness of importance of fruit and vegetable intake for health and well-being	Parental facilitation and direct encouragement	Availability and accessibility of fruit and vegetable at home
Positive taste preferences for different fruits and vegetables	Parental modelling behaviour	Availability and accessibility of fruit and vegetable in the school
Awareness of own fruit and vegetable intake	Peer modelling behaviour	A fruit and vegetable promotion school environment
Awareness of recommended intake levels Self-efficacy and skills for asking for fruit and vegetable Self-efficacy and skills for preparing fruit and vegetable Self-efficacy and skills for obtaining fruit and vegetable Self-efficacy and skills for keeping fruit and vegetable fresh Familiarity with different fruits and vegetables	Teacher support	Neighbourhood support

programme to the end-users and intermediaries. For school-based interventions, this means interaction with pupils, teachers and other school staff, as well as parents [12]. Finally, at step 5, IM focuses on developing a plan for monitoring the process of implementation and evaluation of the programme's efficacy. It is relevant to have in mind this process from the very early phases of programme development, since the proximal programme objectives inspire the evaluation of programme effects. IM has been described in more detail elsewhere [7].

Mapping the Pro Children Intervention

Since the Pro Children Project aimed to develop a school-based intervention applicable across Europe, IM was used to identify intervention methods and strategies valid in different countries, but leaving open the opportunity to further tailor these methods to each separate country's specific relevant features. The needs assessment and steps 1 and 2 were therefore done for all Pro Children countries together, while steps 3 and 4 were partly country specific. Within the present project, these later steps were fully completed for 3 Pro Children countries in which the Pro Children intervention is being tested: Spain, Norway and the Netherlands [4].

The Needs Assessment

Fruit and vegetable consumption is generally regarded as a health-promoting behaviour [13, 14], but intake of this food group is lower than recommended for many European schoolchildren [2]. We therefore started with the identification of important and changeable determinants of fruit and vegetable intakes in children across Europe. This phase was accomplished by means of a literature review of determinant studies, an exploration of important behavioural determinant theories and focus group interviews with children in 6 Pro Children countries [4, 15].

The literature review revealed that determinant studies for fruit and vegetable intakes in schoolchildren have been mostly based on Bandura's [16] Social Cognitive Theory and social-ecological models [11]. These studies indicate that a mixture of environmental and individual factors predict consumption in children, with taste preferences ('liking') and fruit and vegetable availability as possibly the most important determinants, while beliefs about health outcomes were regarded as less important. Parents were identified as important mediators, since they may influence availability as well as act as role models.

The main determinants were categorized as individual, social and environmental factors (table 1). For all 3 of the intervention countries, availability of fruit and vegetable, preferences and taste were expected to be the most important determinants. A general awareness of the importance of fruit and vegetable intake, recommended intake levels and own intake levels were also regarded as important across countries. For Spain, the needs assessment indicated that peer influences played a role regarding fruit consumption while parental modelling behaviour and family food rules influenced vegetable consumption. Skills for preparing fruit and vegetable and asking for fruit and vegetable, and awareness of own fruit and vegetable intake were relevant as well. In the Netherlands, the focus groups revealed that practical barriers and parenting practices were identified as relevant additional determinants [15]. In Norway, the focus groups additionally revealed that children were concerned about hygiene, quality and food safety issues, especially related to fruit and vegetables available at schools. Time constraint during breakfast and the lunch break was perceived as a barrier as well.

Step 1: Define Proximal Programme Objectives

Selection of Performance Objectives

The general behaviour 'children eat more fruits and vegetables' was further specified into the following individual performance objectives: to assess the adequacy of one's own current fruit and vegetable intake; to become familiar with a variety of fruits and vegetables; to develop skills to ask for fruit and vegetable; to develop skills to obtain fruit and vegetable; to develop skills to keep fruit and vegetable fresh; to develop skills to prepare fruit and vegetable. Performance objectives regarding social influences and environmental conditions to be changed were specified as: parents stimulate their children to eat more fruit and vegetable; parents eat fruit and vegetable with their children to act as role models; children taste and eat fruit and vegetable along with peers at school; fruit and vegetable are made better available and accessible for children at home and school.

Selection of Changeable and Important Determinants of Performance Objectives

The potential correlates and determinants of the specified performance objectives were selected based on the literature review, the focus group interviews [15], as well as a concise review of theoretical models that are currently used to describe and explain nutrition behaviours.

Personal determinants included awareness of recommended intake levels and own intake, skills and self-efficacy for obtaining, preparing, asking for and keeping fruit and vegetable, self-evaluation and fruit and vegetable taste preferences. At the social level, determinants considered were peer influences, parental influences as well as social support. Finally, at the environmental level, determinants considered were availability and accessibility of fruit and vegetable at home and at school, social support and school-based social networks.

Identification of the Target Populations

In the Pro Children Project, the target group was already quite narrowly defined, i.e. 10- to 13-year-old schoolchildren. These children were identified as the ultimate target population for the intervention. Parents and school staff were further target populations since the selection of determinants revealed that these intermediary actors were needed to improve the children's fruit and vegetable environment [12].

Define Learning and Change Objectives

The completion of step 1 was done in a modified way: a two-day workshop was organized at one of the Pro Children centres for all Pro Children staff involved in the intervention development and implementation in January 2003. A matrix was developed by combining the performance objectives and relevant determinants (tables 2, 3).

Step 2: Select Suitable Theoretical Methods and Practical Strategies

Subsequently, we had brainstorm sessions to select suitable methods and strategies to reach the learning objectives that were regarded as realistic within the Pro Children context. The selection of useful theoretical methods included information transfer, role modelling, skill building, skill transfer, self-assessment and feedback, problem solving, goal setting, active learning, incentives, social support, guided practice and reinforcement [8, 17–21].

Evidence for the effectiveness of school-based nutrition education programmes also suggests that the following features contribute to successful nutrition education: the use of theory-driven educational strategies directly relevant to a behavioural focus; devotion of adequate time and intensity to the intervention; family involvement, particularly in programmes for younger children; incorporation of self-evaluation or self-assessment and feedback in interventions for older children; interventions in the school environment and interventions in the larger community which can enhance school nutrition and health education [17, 18]. Schools provide a well-established setting for implementing health promotion interventions aimed at children and their important others [20–23].

At a very early stage of the intervention development, we conducted a feasibility study in order to identify similarities and differences among intervention sites, strengths and weaknesses in school systems and the potential of available resources. The feasibility study explored the school systems and other potential organizations or settings relevant for the intervention; the way nutrition education is considered in schools in each intervention site, how much effort is dedicated to that,

Table 2. Matrix of learning objectives for schoolchildren in the Pro Children intervention arranged by determinants: personal determinants

Performance objectives	Personal determinants				
	awareness	skills	self-efficacy	self-evaluation	preferences/taste
To assess adequacy of one's own current fruit and vegetable intake	Children are aware of importance of fruit and vegetable intake for health and well-being	Children can complete a computer-based fruit and vegetable test		Children complete a computer-based fruit and vegetable test	
	Children are aware of recommended intake levels	Children can read and understand a feedback report		Children read and understand a tailored feedback report	
	Children know what is a portion of fruit and a portion of vegetables	Children develop skills to identify what is a portion of fruit and a portion of vegetables		Children set goals for increased consumption	Children taste a variety of fruits and vegetables at home Children taste a variety of fruits and vegetables at school
	Children know what a fruit juice is and what is not				Children taste a variety of fruit juices at school
	Children are aware of own intake			Children experience success in eating more fruit and vegetable per day	
To become familiar with a variety of fruit and vegetable	Children are aware of what influences their fruit and vegetable preferences	Children are able to describe taste and other characteristics of fruit and vegetable	Children feel confident they can try fruit and vegetable they have not tasted before	Children set goals for increased consumption	Children become familiar with a variety of fruits and vegetables and try kinds not tested before
To ask for fruit and vegetable in different settings		Children develop skills to ask for fruit and vegetable at home Children develop skills to ask for fruit and vegetable in a variety of settings	Children feel confident they can ask for fruit and vegetable at home	Children set goals for increased consumption	
To be able to obtain fruit and vegetable in different situations	Children identify different places where they can get fruit and vegetable Children identify a variety of fruit and vegetable	Children develop skills to get/ buy fruit and vegetable Children are involved in buying fruit and vegetable	Children feel confident they can get fruit and vegetable at home	Children set goals for increased consumption	Children taste 'new' fruits and vegetables
To be able to keep fruit and vegetable fresh and attractive	Children are aware of how fruit and vegetable are best preserved Children identify fruit and vegetable safety issues	Children develop skills to get, keep and prepare fruit and vegetable considering food safety	Children feel confident they can keep safely fruit and vegetable		
To be able to prepare fruit and vegetable	Children are aware that fruit and vegetable can be prepared in many different ways	Children develop skills to prepare fruit and vegetable	Children feel confident they can prepare fruit and vegetable with some help at home		Children are exposed to different preparations based on fruit and vegetable at home Children are exposed to different preparations based on fruit and vegetable at school

Table 3. Matrix of change objectives for external determinants in the Pro Children intervention

Performance objectives	Social and environmental determinants				
	peer influences	parental influences	availability and accessibility	neighbourhood support	a fruit and vegetable promotion school environment
To assess adequacy of one's own current fruit and vegetable intake	Children complete a computer-based fruit and vegetable test at school with their peers	Children read tailored feedback report with their parents Parents complete a computer-based fruit and vegetable test Parents can read and understand a tailored feedback report		Local media report on fruit and vegetable facts and issues	
To become familiar with a variety of fruit and vegetable	Children taste a variety of fruit and vegetable with their peers Children taste a variety of fruit juices with their peers Peers act as role models eating and tasting fruit and vegetable together	Children taste a variety of fruit and vegetable with their parents Parents act as role models for children eating fruit and vegetable with them	Parents increase availability and accessibility of fruit and vegetable at home Schools cooperate to increase availability of fruit and vegetable in school		School project committees/school health programme and other health-related bodies support increased availability of fruit and vegetable at school
To ask for fruit and vegetable in different settings		Parents stimulate their children to eat more fruit and vegetable	Children find fruit and vegetable at school Children find fruit and vegetable at home		School health programme reinforces children's demand of fruit and vegetable
To be able to obtain fruit and vegetable in different situations	Children share shopping experiences	Children buy fruit and vegetable with their parents		Grocery stores highlight importance of fruit and vegetable	
To be able to keep safely fruit and vegetable	Children share experiences in keeping fruit and vegetable	Children keep fruit and vegetable at home with their parents			
To be able to prepare fruit and vegetable	Children share experiences in preparing fruit and vegetable	Children prepare fruit and vegetable at home with their parents	Increases availability and access of fruit and vegetable at home		

which teacher or any other person is responsible for nutrition education in schools; whether it is considered as a separate subject in the curriculum; possible school food service and other possibilities children may find in the school to get food; existing school food policies or norms regarding the provision of food or access to food in schools; possibilities to organize out-of-the classroom activities in schools; continuing education for teachers; existing school health committees or potential for creating them; availability of computer facilities and internet access in schools. All this information was collected from existing documents and personal interviews with heads of schools, curriculum developers and other school staff in each country.

Step 3: Design a Programme Plan

A further brainstorm session was held to identify existing intervention tools and activities in the 3 intervention countries that fitted the methods and learning objectives and that were applicable given the time, setting and financial restraints of the Pro Children Project. Next we decided on necessary adjustments of existing tools, for example in order to make tools developed in one country applicable in the other Pro Children intervention countries. Subsequently, we considered the cells in the matrices (tables 2, 3) that were not yet covered by an existing intervention tool, to explore if new tools could be developed for those cells.

Finally, theoretically similar but culturally relevant interventions were developed to be implemented and evaluated in Norway, the Netherlands and Spain during 2 school years. The programme is meant to be applicable in all Pro Children countries with few adaptations. The Pro Children programme was arranged into three different components: (a) *classroom component,* namely school-based educational material for children consisting of a set of worksheets with guided activities for the classroom and out-of-the classroom; a computer-tailored instrument developed to be used by children at school and a teachers' manual; (b) *school component (school environment),* with provision of fruit and vegetable in the schools as the main element, either as free in-school distribution, a subscription programme, or as part of school meals; building of school project committees as a supportive structure was encouraged as a means of stimulating participation of all school members in the project; parents, pupils, teachers, school food service personnel, school health people and other interested members in the community were invited to be members of the school project committee; (c) *family component,* consisting of active parent involvement in the children's homework worksheets. Parents were informed about these homework tasks by specially designed letters. Additionally, an existing Internet-based computer-tailored tool [24] to provide parents with personalized feedback on the intake levels and perceived barriers was adjusted and used in the present project, and 5 newsletters for parents were developed that included a variety of information on fruit and vegetable, announcements about ongoing activities in the Pro Children programme and tips for parents to encourage their children to eat more fruit and vegetable. The 3 intervention sites shared a common outline for each newsletter, but added country-relevant information. The computer-tailored tool and the newsletters were also available via the Pro Children website [25]. Additionally, this website was used as a communication and exchange tool with participating schools.

Each intervention site added one optional component, either involvement of the media, school health services or grocery stores [26]. The objectives of these additional components were to encourage community participation in the Pro Children Project and to stimulate a social environment supportive to children eating more fruit and vegetable. In the Netherlands, the media was used to raise project awareness and active commitment to the project. In Spain, school health services were used to foster school food policies; counsel students on eating fruit and vegetable in the course of routine health screening exams; providing advise to families on eating an adequate amount of fruit and vegetable and reminding them about their supportive role during routine interviews. In Norway, grocery stores were used to provide basic information on fruit and vegetable to consumers and thus contributing to raising awareness.

Professional advice from designers guided the final layout of all educational materials. Designers also depicted a logo and a Pro Children poster. All educational materials, including the logo, poster, worksheets, computer tailoring and school manual, were pretested in the context of personal interviews with parents, teachers and school staff and by means of focus groups with children. Additionally, the main educational materials were pretested in classrooms. The goal of the pretesting was to find out whether the materials were attractive, personally relevant, easy enough to understand and easy to use. Table 4 shows the selected strategies related to learning objectives and modifiable determinants.

Step 4: Adoption and Implementation Plan

A plan for implementation and adoption of the programme was designed including implementation objectives, methods and strategies. Adequate time, intensity of the intervention, resources, as well as the provision of suitable materials and teacher training opportunities are essential for successful implementation. The involvement of teachers and children in the development phase improved the chances for adoption and implementation, and the pretesting of the materials allowed for further improvement. Additionally, we used teacher training sessions supplemented with comprehensive teacher and school manuals to promote adequate adoption and effective implementation of the programme.

Step 5: Monitoring and Evaluation Plan

From the very early stages in programme development, formative, process and outcome evaluation plans were designed. Formative evaluation was used to guard IM steps 3 and 4. The process evaluation protocol guided the investigation of the degree of programme implementation across the 3 intervention sites. The protocol included monitoring of the intervention delivery and perceived satisfaction and evaluation of the programme by key actors. Process evaluation was based on observations, face-to-face interviews with school staff, focus groups with children, and self-administered questionnaires for children, staff and parents. Additionally, teachers were asked to keep a logbook when performing each activity in the classroom. The information collected in the process evaluation was used to identify facilitating factors and barriers for implementation to enable further improvement before broader dissemination.

Table 4. Selected educational strategies related to learning objectives and modifiable determinants in the Pro Children intervention

Learning objectives	Determinant						
	availability	awareness	preferences/ taste	peer influences	parental influences	skills	
						prepare	ask/obtain
Children are aware of importance of fruit and vegetable intake for health and well-being		Education worksheet-guided activity					
Children know recommendation		CT feedback Education worksheet-guided activity					
Children know what a fruit juice is and what is not		Education worksheet on label reading	Taste-testing activity at school				
Fruit and vegetable is an issue for children		Education worksheet-guided activity CT feedback		Web-based international discussion forum			
Children find fruit and vegetable at school	School fruit (fruit break)			Eat fruit and vegetable together in class	Parents give fruit and vegetable to children to bring to school		
Children find fruit and vegetable at home		Newsletter for parents			Newsletter for parents	Preparing fruit and vegetable at home Education work-sheet-guided activity	CT encour-agement to ask for fruit and vegetable
Children are exposed to different fruits and vegetables	School fruit (fruit break)		Fruit taste-testing activity at school	Peer leading activity	Vegetables taste testing game at home with parents		
Children are involved in buying fruit and vegetable	Children buy fruit and vegeta-ble with parents (homework)						Quality and safety education worksheet
Children taste 'new' fruit and vegetable			Fruit taste-testing game	Eating fruit together in class	Vegetables taste testing game at home with parents	Recipe competition Preparing fruit and vegetable at home Education work-sheet-guided activity	
Make children aware of what influences their preferences		Peer leading activity Education worksheet-guided activity	Education worksheet-guided activity	Group discussion Web-based discus-sion forum Educa-tion worksheet-guided activity			
Children are aware of own intake		CT feedback Education worksheet					
Children know how to prepare fruit and vegetable		Newsletter for parents			Preparing fruit and vegetable at home	Education work-sheet-guided activity	
Children set goals for increased consumption Parents are aware of own behaviour		CT feedback Education worksheet Newsletter for parents			Parental support Self-test, CT feedback		Education worksheet

CT = Computer-tailored feedback.

The outcome evaluation plan was intended to guide the assessment of the effects of the Pro Children intervention on fruit and vegetable intakes, performance objectives and determinants [4].

Discussion

Although applying the IM protocol to develop the Pro Children intervention required time and effort, it helped us to carefully consider each decision in the intervention development and implementation preparation. It further strongly encouraged using evidence-based and theory-driven intervention methods, strategies and materials. Furthermore, IM helped us to systematically get input from different actors, such as programme developers, users and the target population, thus ensuring participation and involvement of key actors in all developmental stages of the programme. As a result, the programme was tailored to the specific needs and characteristics of participants as well as to available resources and skills of the main actors.

IM was also useful for planning the evaluation, since we used our inventory of performance and learning objectives to specify intermediary outcome indicators and to develop the survey instruments. We thus included outcome indicators at the behaviour and determinant levels, and at the individual and environmental levels.

Since application of IM completely according to the instruction given by the originators [7] takes more time than was available within the Pro Children time frame, we used a modified version of the IM protocol to speed up the process. We combined steps 1 and 2 when developing matrices, although the process of formulating explicit learning and change objectives was included, and we restricted the amount and complexity of matrices that guide decision making according to IM.

Using IM means that an intervention is not well laid out at the start of a project. This means that funding agencies need to decide on such projects without detailed information on the intervention contents, but should instead rely on the description of the development process. In the Pro Children example, we should acknowledge the courage of the project reviewers and the European Commission to approve and grant the project despite the absence of a clear-cut intervention plan, having confidence in the IM-driven careful intervention development plan.

Among the other potential strengths of the Pro Children intervention, we would like to stress that it was aimed at both the individual and the environmental level, including suggestions for organizational change such as building school project committees and changes in school policies like creating the fruit break. The Pro Children intervention encouraged active participation in learning processes and family support. Some of the learning methods make use of new technologies, such as computer-tailored tools and the website, which also served as a practical tool for cross-topic teaching experiences, involving English teachers, technology teachers and/or the usual classroom teacher.

In conclusion, the Pro Children intervention was carefully developed based on the IM protocol that resulted in a comprehensive school-based fruit and vegetable promotion programme. This programme, which uses a common standard intervention programme but at the same time allows fine-tuning to country-specific needs, is now available in 4 different languages, i.e. Norwegian, Dutch, Spanish and Basque. It has been implemented and is tested in 3 European countries.

Acknowledgement

This study is being carried out with financial support from the Commission of the European Communities, specific RTD programme 'Quality of Life and Management of Living Resources', QLK1-2001-00547 'Promoting and Sustaining Health through Increased Vegetable and Fruit Consumption among European Schoolchildren' (Pro Children). The study does not necessarily reflect the Commission's views and in no way anticipates the Commission's future policy in this area.

References

1 Currie C: Young People's Health in Context: Health Behaviour in School-Aged Children (HBSC) Study: International Report from the 2001/2002 Survey. Copenhagen, WHO Regional Office for Europe, 2004.

2 Yngve A, Wolf A, Poortvliet E, Elmadfa I, Brug J, Ehrenblad B, Franchini B, Haraldsdóttir J, Krølner R, Maes L, Pérez-Rodrigo C, Sjöström M, Thórsdóttir I, Klepp K-I: Fruit and vegetable intake in a sample of 11-year-old children in 9 European countries: the Pro Children cross-sectional survey. Ann Nutr Metab 2005;49:236–245.

3 Lien N, Lytle LA, Klepp KI: Stability in consumption of fruit, vegetables, and sugary foods in a cohort from age 14 to age 21. Prev Med 2001;33:217–226.

4 Klepp K-I, Pérez-Rodrigo C, De Bourdeaudhuij I, Due P, Elmadfa I, Haraldsdóttir J, König J, Sjöström M, Thórsdóttir I, de Almeida MDV, Yngve A, Brug J: Promoting fruit and vegetable consumption among European schoolchildren: rationale, conceptualization and design of the Pro Children Project. Ann Nutr Metab 2005;49:212–220.

5 Green LW, Kreuter MW: Health Promotion Planning: An Educational and Ecological Approach, ed 3. Mountain View, Mayfield, 1999.

6 McKenzie JF, Smeltzer JL: Planning, Implementing, and Evaluating Health Promotion Programs: A Primer, ed 3. Boston, Allyn and Bacon, 2001.

7 Bartholomew KL, Parcel GS, Kok G, Gottlieb NH: Intervention Mapping: Designing Theory- and Evidence-Based Health Promotion Programs. Mountain View, Mayfield, 2001.

8 Kok G, Schaalma H, Ruiter R, Empelen P van, Brug J: Intervention mapping: a protocol for applying health psychology theory to prevention programmes. J Health Psychol 2004;9: 85–89.

9 Brug J, Oenema A, Ferreira I: Theory, evidence and Intervention Mapping to improve behavioural nutrition and physical activity interventions. Int J Behav Nutr Phys Act 2005; 2:2.

10 Cullen KW, Baranowski T, Owens E, Marsh T, Rittenberry L, de Moor C: Availability, accessibility, and preferences for fruit, 100% fruit juice, and vegetables influence children's dietary behaviour. Health Educ Behav 2003;30: 615–626.

11 Baranowski T, Cullen KW, Nicklas T, Thompson D, Baranowski J: Are current health behavioural change models helpful in guiding prevention of weight gain efforts? Obes Res 2003; 11(suppl):23S–43S.

12 French SA, Stables G: Environmental interventions to promote vegetable and fruit consumption among youth in school settings. Prev Med 2003;37:593–610.

13 Van Duyn MA, Pivonka E: Overview of the health benefits of fruit and vegetable consumption for the dietetics professional: selected literature. J Am Diet Assoc 2000;100:1511–1521.

14 Hung HC, Joshipura KJ, Jiang R, Hu FB, Hunter D, Smith-Warner SA, Colditz GA, Rosner B, Spiegelman D, Willett WC: Fruit and vegetable intake and risk of major chronic disease. J Natl Cancer Inst 2004;96:1577–1584.

15 Wind M, Bobelijn K, De Bourdeaudhuij I, Klepp K-I, Brug J: A qualitative exploration of determinants of fruit and vegetable intake among 10- and 11-year-old schoolchildren in the Low Countries. Ann Nutr Metab 2005;49:228–235.

16 Bandura A: Self-Efficacy: The Exercise of Control. New York, Freeman and Company, 1997.

17 Hoelscher DM, Evans A, Parcel GS, Kelder SH: Designing effective nutrition interventions for adolescents. J Am Diet Assoc 2002; 102(suppl 3):s52–s63.

18 Contento I, Balch GI, Bronner YL, Lytle LA, Maloney SK, Olson CM, Swadener SS: The effectiveness of nutrition education and implications for nutrition education policy, programs and research: a review of research. J Nutr Educ 1995;27:279–418.

19 Cullen KW, Zakeri I, Pryor EW, Baranowski T, Baranowski J, Watson K: Goal setting is differentially related to change in fruit, juice, and vegetable consumption among fourth-grade children. Health Educ Behav 2004;31:258–269.

20 Wechsler H, Devereaux RS, Davis M, Collins J: Using the school environment to promote physical activity and healthy eating. Prev Med 2000;31:S121–S137.

21 Perry C, Bishop BD, Taylor CA, Davis M, Story M, Gray C, Bishop SC, Warren Mays R, Lytle LA, Harnack L: A randomized school trial of environmental strategies to encourage fruit and vegetable consumption among children. Health Educ Behav 2004;31:63–76.

22 Perez-Rodrigo C, Aranceta J: Nutrition education in schools: experiences and challenges. Eur J Clin Nutr 2003;57(suppl 1):S82–S85.

23 Reynolds KD, Pass MA, Galvin M, Winnail SD, Harrington KF, DiClemente RJ. Schools as a setting for health promotion and disease prevention; in Raczynski JM, DiCelemente RJ (eds): Handbook of Health Promotion and Disease Prevention. New York, Kluwer Academic/Plenum Publishers, 1999, pp 397–425.

24 Oenema A, Tan F, Brug J: Short-term effect of a web-based computer-tailored nutrition intervention: main effects and mediators. Ann Behav Med 2005;29:54–63.

25 Pro Children Consortium: The Pro Children Project. www.univie.ac.at/prochildren/ (accessed February 10, 2005).

26 Story M, Neumark-Sztainer D, French S: Individual and environmental influences on adolescent eating behaviours. J Am Diet Assoc 2002;102(3 suppl):S40–S51.

Author Index Vol. 49, No. 4, 2005

Annals of
Nutrition & Metabolism

Subject Index Vol. 49, No. 4, 2005

KARGER
Fax +41 61 306 12 34
E-Mail karger@karger.ch
www.karger.com

Accessible online at:
www.karger.com/anm

The Official *FENS* Calendar

Ann Nutr Metab 2005;49:279–280

This section provides information about the meetings and events of all FENS member societies. The list of events is by no means inclusive, and the publisher is not responsible for any data given.

Event	Place/Date	Organizing Society	Contact for information	Web-Site
Aktuelle Aspekte der Ernährungsbildung und – beratung	Paderborn / Germany September 29-30, 2005	German Nutrition Society (DGE)	DGE Department of Public Relations Godesberger Allee 18 D-53175 Bonn Tel.: +49 228 3776 600 Fax: +49 228 3776 800	www.dge.de
Macro- and micronutrients – a source of health National conference with international participation	Jurata / Poland September 6-9, 2005	Polish Society of Nutritional Sciences	Polish Society of Nutritional Sciences Dept. of Human Nutrition SGGW PL-02-787 Warsaw Tel.: +48 22 843 83 15 Fax: + 48 22 847 00 12 e-mail: j.bertrandt@wihe.waw.pl	
European Childhood Obesity Group (ECOG) Childhood Obesity: New Insights and Consequences	Vienna / Austria September 29-October 2, 2005	Österreichisches Akademisches Institut für Ernährungsmedizin	Ivana Gründler Projektmanagement Österr. Akad. Institut für Ernährungsmedizin Neulerchenfelderstr. 6-8 A-1160 Wien Tel: + 43 1 402 64 72 Fax: +43 1 402 92 22 e-mail: office@oeaie.org	www.oeaie.org
Facts and illusions in human nutrition: phosphorus in human nutrition – advantages and threat. National conference and celebration of the 25 anniversary of the Society	Warsaw / Poland October 21, 2005	Polish Society of Nutritional Sciences	Polish Society of Nutritional Sciences Attn.: Prof. Dr. hab. Anna Gronowska-Senger Dept. of Human Nutrition SGGW PL-02-787 Warsaw Tel.: +48 22 843 83 15 Fax: + 48 22 847 00 12 e-mail: senger@alpha.sggw.waw.pl	

KARGER
Fax + 41 61 306 12 34
E-Mail karger@karger.ch
www.karger.com

Accessible online at:
www.karger.com/anm

Children's Nutrition and Food for Adolescents	Vienna / Austria November 17-18, 2005	Austrian Nutrition Society	Mag. Alexandra Hofer ÖGE-Geschaftsstelle Zaunergasse 1-3 A-1030 Vienna Tel. +43 1 714 71 93 Fax + +43 1 718 61 46 e-mail: info@oege.at	www.oege.at
ÖAK-Diplom Ernährungsmedizin Ausbildungszyklen 2006	Vienna / Austria 2006 (for exact dates please see online)	Österreichisches Akademisches Institut für Ernährungsmedizin	Ivana Gründler Projektmanagement Österr. Akad. Institut für Ernährungsmedizin Neulerchenfelderstr. 6-8 A-1160 Wien Tel: + 43 1 402 64 72 Fax: +43 1 402 92 22 e-mail: office@oeaie.org	www.oeaie.org

European Academy of Nutritional Sciences

EANS Society News

EANS Officials 2005 (Interim)

President:
Prof. P.J. Aggett

Vice-Presidents:
Prof. Carlo Agostoni
Dr. Carmen Pérez Rodrigo

Secretary General:
Dr. Jean-Michel Antoine

Treasurer:
Dr. Pierre Guesry

Website Committee:
Prof. Dr. P.J. Aggett

Website:
www.eans.net

EANS Secretariat:
E-mail: info@eans.net

Mission

EANS is an association of individual nutritional scientists sharing the following aims:

- to be the custodian of the quality of the European nutritional science
- to support the high quality education of young nutritional scientists
- to create a platform for discussing, summarizing and communicating important nutritional issues

To achieve these aims EANS will:

- encourage and support the organization of high quality symposia and workshops within Europe. EANS patronage is a mark of quality
- encourage and support its members to play an active role in public debates on nutrition
- encourage its members to be active in training programmes for young scientists, both in scientific and communicative fields

The strength of EANS is the quality of its members. The membership selection procedures ensure, that this will remain so.

Membership

EANS Secretariat
Dr. Jean-Michel Antoine
Danone Vitapole
Route Départementale 128
F–91767 Palaiseau Cedex (France)
E-Mail jean-michel.antoine@danone.com

Next Meeting

EANS Annual Conference
'Nutrition and Childhood,
Nutrition and Elderly'
Bilbao, November 2–3, 2006

KARGER

Fax +41 61 306 12 34
E-Mail karger@karger.ch
www.karger.com

Accessible online at:
www.karger.com/anm

KI 04681

European **A**cademy *of* **N**utritional **S**ciences

EANS Membership Application Form

Membership of the *European Academy of Nutritional Sciences*:
Active members of the Academy (yearly fee EUR 20.–): eligible as active members of the Academy are individuals, who have distinguished themselves in sciences related to nutrition.

***EANS* application procedures:**
Candidates may apply individually for membership by completing the application form below or online at: **www.eans.net**. A one-page CV and a list of your 10 most important publications (title and reference) must be included in your application. When the Secretary concludes that all the formal criteria have been met, he will then ask the Presidium for the applicant to be presented for election to the General Assembly.

Application form:

Name: ____________________

Company/Institution: ____________________

____

Address: ____________________

Postal code: __________ City: __________

Country: __________

Tel.: __________ Fax: __________

E-Mail: ____________________

2 main areas of expertise: ____________________

Additional comments: ____________________

Please submit this form to:
EANS Secretariat
Dr. Jean-Michel Antoine
Danone Vitapole
Route Départementale 128
F–91767 Palaiseau Cedex (France)
E-Mail jean-michel.antoine@danone.com

KARGER

Fax +41 61 306 12 34
E-Mail karger@karger.ch
www.karger.com

Accessible online at:
www.karger.com/anm

KI 04682

The European NutriGenomics Organisation

The European Nutrigenomics Organisation (NuGO) – Linking Genomics, Nutrition and Health Research

Leading centres in nutritional research from across Europe have come together to create a Network of Excellence, the European Nutrigenomics Organisation, linking genomics, nutrition and health research. Led by Dr. Ben van Ommen, NuGO has been awarded €17.3 million over a period of 6 years and currently has 22 partners from 10 EU member states.

The network is a virtual centre of excellence to integrate and develop genomic technologies for the benefit of European nutritional science, to facilitate the application of these technologies in nutritional research and train a new generation of scientists to use them. More specifically, the aims are to:

- Strengthen the European scientific and technological excellence in nutrigenomics by bringing together the critical mass of resources and expertise needed to offer leadership in this rapidly developing field
- Define individual response to nutrients and refine the requirements for population sub-groups based on genetic variations (nutrigenetics), sex, and the different life stages
- Determine the relative health benefits and risks of food compounds for different population sub-groups and improve public health
- Spread excellence in nutrigenomics beyond the partnership through training, sharing of methods and facilities, dissemination and exploitation, and enter into dialogue with stakeholder groups
- Support the competitive arm of the European food industry, facilitating its growth as a knowledge-based business, with a view to evidence-based healthier food production
- Promote understanding in the ethical, social, legal, economical and scientific issues of concern in nutrigenomics

Activities

The **Integrating Activities** will harmonise, stimulate and facilitate new technology, informatics and systems for common use, and underpin research activities. Work packages are:

- Nutrigenomics technology standardisation and innovation – Ruan Elliott
- Genomics methods for nutritional studies in humans and model systems – John Mathers
- Bioinformatics and nutritional systems biology – Rob Stierum
- Information systems and databases – Heiner Boeing

The **Joint Research Activities** plan to exploit the technological and scientific innovations in a number of key areas of nutrition and health research as well as consolidate the research effort in Europe. Work packages are:

- Gut health and function – Piero Dolaro
- Metabolic health – Helen Roche
- Life stage nutrition – Harry McArdle
- Risk benefit evaluation – Jaap Keijer

The **Spreading of Excellence Activities** will build upon the acquired knowledge, sharing it with stakeholder groups including researchers, industry, society and healthcare. Work packages are:

- Training – Wilma Steegenga
- Communication – Catherine Reynolds
- Nutrigenomics and society – Christien Enzing
- SME recruitement and management – Regine Schreiner

NuGO Partners

European Molecular Biology Laboratory, European Bioinformatics Institute, UK; German Institute of Human Nutrition (DIfE), Germany; Institute of Food Research (IFR), UK; Lund University, Sweden; Maastricht University, The Netherlands; National Institute of Health and Medical Research (INSERM), France; National Institute of Public Health and the Environment (RIVM), The Netherlands; RIKILT – Institute of Food Safety, The Netherlands; Rowett Research Institute, Aberdeen, UK; Technische Universität München (TUM) – Nutrigenomics Center, Germany; The Jagiellonian University Medical College, Poland; TNO Nutrition and Food Research, The Netherlands; Topshare International BV, Wageningen, The Netherlands (SME); Trinity College Dublin (TCD), Ireland; University College Cork – National University of Ireland, Ireland; University of Firenze, Italy; University of Newcastle, UK; University of Oslo, Norway; University of Reading, Centre for Integrated Nutritional Genomics, UK; University of the Balearic Islands, Spain; University of Ulster, Coleraine, UK; Wageningen University, The Netherlands.

Further information can be obtained from:

Dr. Siân Astley
NuGO Communications Manager
Institute of Food Research
Norwich Research Park
Colney, Norwich NR4 7UA (UK)
Tel.: +44 1603 255219
Fax: +44 1603 255168
E-Mail: sian.astley@bbsrc.ac.uk
www.nugo.org
CT-2004-505944

Guidelines for Authors

Annals of
Nutrition & Metabolism

Submission

The journal consists of the following sections:

1. Editorials
2. Review Articles
3. Original Papers
4. Case Reports
5. Announcements

Manuscripts written in English are considered and should be sent to:

Prof. Dr. I. Elmadfa
Institute of Nutritional Sciences
University of Vienna
Althanstrasse 14
A-1090 Vienna (Austria)
Tel. +43 1 4277 54901
Fax +43 1 4277 9549
E-Mail ernaehrungswissenschaften@univie.ac.at

Manuscripts should be submitted in triplicate (with three sets of illustrations of which one is an original; final high-resolution pictures need only be sent after acceptance of the paper) together with a soft copy on disc. **The manuscript should match the electronic file exactly.** For details please refer to: www.karger.com/electronic_submission. Editorial work and copy-editing will be executed from the electronic version of your manuscript.

Conditions

All manuscripts are subject to editorial review. Manuscripts are received with the explicit understanding that they are not under simultaneous consideration by any other publication. Submission of an article for publication implies transfer of the copyright from the author to the publisher upon acceptance. Accepted papers become the permanent property of 'Annals of Nutrition and Metabolism' and may not be reproduced by any means, in whole or in part, without the written consent of the publisher. It is the author's responsibility to obtain permission to reproduce illustrations, tables, etc. from other publications.

Special Requirements

1. Investigations Involving Human Subjects: 'Annals of Nutrition and Metabolism' requires that investigations performed on human subjects have the prior approval of the institutional committee on human experimentation. Authors are required to submit a signed statement as to the date and details of the appropriate review. In countries where such mechanisms for approval do not exist, authors are required to submit a signed statement that the research was carried out in accordance with the Helsinki Declaration. A similar assurance is required to document that animal experimentation was performed under appropriate circumstances.
2. Statement for Authors Submitting Original Research or Case Reports: 'The enclosed manuscript ... (Title) ... has been approved by me as well as by the responsible authorities at the institute where the work has been carried out. I certify that none of the material in this manuscript has been published previously in any form and that none of this material is currently under consideration for publication elsewhere. This includes symposia and proceedings of meetings and preliminary publications of any kind except an abstract of 400 words or less.' (To be signed by all authors.)
3. The undersigned also confirm that they qualify for (co-)authorship according to the 'Uniform Requirements for Manuscripts' published in the guidelines of the 'International Committee of Medical Journal Editors' in 1988 as follows: Authorship credit should be based only on substantial contributions to (a) conception and design, or analysis and interpretation of data; (b) drafting the article or revising it critically for important intellectual content; and (c) final approval of the version to be published. Conditions (a), (b), and (c) must all be met. Participation solely in the acquisition of funding or the collection of data does not justify authorship. General supervision of the research group is also not sufficient for authorship. Any part of an article critical to its main conclusions must be the responsibility of at least one author. Persons who have contributed intellectually to the article but whose contributions do not justify authorship may be named and their particular contribution described in the 'Acknowledgements'. Such persons must give their permission to be named.

Arrangement

Title page: The first page of each paper should indicate the title, the authors' names, the institute where the work was conducted, and a short title for use as running head. NB: Authors wishing to preserve the phonetic meaning of diacritics (PubMed reduces diacritics to their root characters) must spell their names accordingly when submitting manuscripts (e.g. Müller should be Mueller).

Full address: The exact postal address of the corresponding author complete with postal code must be given at the bottom of the title page. Please also supply phone and fax numbers, as well as e-mail address.

Key words: For indexing purposes, a list of 3–10 key words in English is essential.

Abstract: Each paper needs an abstract of up to 200 words. It should be structured as follows:

Background/Aims:	What is the major problem that prompted the study?
Methods:	How was the study performed?
Results:	Most important findings?
Conclusion:	Most important conclusion?

Methods: The reader should be able to follow the methods by which the results were obtained, but there is no need for detailed descriptions unless of a genuine innovation.

Results: The results should be described precisely and must be separated from the discussion.

Discussion: The discussion should be confined to the interpretation of the results and should not consist of a repetition of them.

Footnotes: Avoid footnotes.

Tables and illustrations: Tables and illustrations (both numbered in Arabic numerals) should be prepared on separate pages. Tables require a heading and figures a legend, also prepared on a separate page. For the reproduction of illustrations, only good drawings and original photographs can be accepted; negatives or photocopies cannot be used. Due to technical reasons, figures with a screen background should not be submitted. When possible, group several illustrations in one block for reproduction (max. size 180 × 223 mm) or provide crop marks. On the back of each illustration, indicate its number, the author's name, and 'top' with a soft pencil. Electronically submitted b/w halftone and color illustrations must have a final resolution of 300 dpi after scaling, line drawings one of 800–1,200 dpi.

Color illustrations: Up to 6 color illustrations per page can be integrated within the text at the special price of CHF/USD 660.00 per page. Color illustrations are reproduced at the author's expense.

References: In the text, identify references by Arabic numerals [in square brackets]. Material submitted for publication but not yet accepted should be noted as 'unpublished data' and not be included in the reference list. The list of references should include only those publications which are cited in the text. Do not alphabetize; number references in the order in which they are first mentioned in the text. The surnames of the authors followed by initials should be given. There should be no punctuation other than a comma to separate the authors. Preferably, please cite all authors. Abbreviate journal names according to the Index Medicus system. (Also see International Committee of Medical Journal Editors: Uniform requirements for manuscripts submitted to biomedical journals. N Engl J Med 1997;336:309–315. www.icmje.org)

Digital Object Identifier (DOI)
S. Karger Publishers supports DOIs as unique identifiers for articles. A DOI number will be printed on the title page of each article. DOIs can be useful in the future for identifying and citing articles published online without volume or issue information. More information can be found at www.doi.org.

Examples
(a) Papers published in periodicals: Chatel J-M, Bernard H, Orson FM: Isolation and characterization of two complete Ara h 2 isoforms cDNA. Int Arch Allergy Immunol 2003;131:14–18.
(b) Papers published only with DOI numbers: Theoharides TC, Boucher W, Spear K: Serum interleukin-6 reflects disease severity and osteoporosis in mastocytosis patients. Int Arch Allergy Immunol DOI: 10.1159/000063858.
(c) Monographs: Matthews DE, Farewell VT: Using and Understanding Medical Statistics, ed 3, revised. Basel, Karger, 1996.
(d) Edited books: DuBois RN: Cyclooxygenase-2 and colorectal cancer; in Dannenberg AJ, Dubois RN (eds): COX-2. Prog Exp Tum Res. Basel, Karger, 2003, vol 37, pp 124–137.

Page charges

There are no page charges for papers of 3 or fewer printed pages (including tables, illustrations and references). Each additional complete or partial page is charged to the author at CHF/USD 275.00. The allotted size of a paper is equal to approx. 10 manuscript pages (including tables, illustrations and references).

Proofs

Unless indicated otherwise, proofs are sent to the first-named author and should be returned with the least possible delay. Alterations made in proofs, other than the correction of printer's errors, are charged to the author.

Reprints

Order forms and a price list are sent with the proofs. Orders submitted after the issue is printed are subject to considerably higher prices.

KARGER

Fax +41 61 306 12 34
E-Mail karger@karger.ch
www.karger.com

The Guidelines for Authors are available at:
www.karger.com/anm_Guidelines

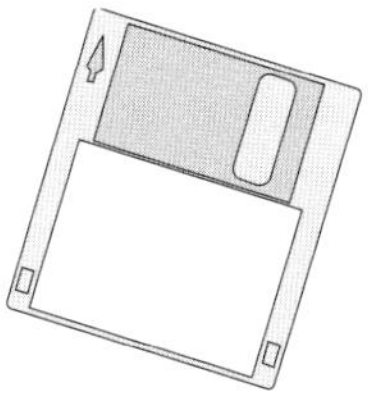

Disk Submission

A **comprehensive version** of these guidelines for the **submission of manuscripts and illustrations on disk** can be accessed online under **www.karger.com/disksubmission** or requested as a leaflet from the editorial department.

Please follow the general rules on style and arrangement in the **'Guidelines for Authors'** of the journal. Submit a **double-spaced printout** of your manuscript matching the file on disk exactly.

Technical Information
Store only data pertinent to this manuscript. Include your fonts (screen and printer fonts for Macintosh). For a **text only** manuscript, use a 3.5-inch disk. For **text and illustrations,** use 3.5 or 5.25 Magneto Optical Disc; CD-ROM (DOS or hybrid); iomega Zip/DOS (100 MB), or 44 MB, 88 MB or 200 MB SyQuest. Compress extensive data using ZIP format.

Data Description
Label your disk with the **title of the journal or book** for which it is submitted; a **short version** of the paper's title; your **name,** postal and e-mail address, fax and phone number; **hard- and software** used, including the version; and the **complete list of the file names.** File names consist of eight characters before the dot identifying the file and three characters after the dot identifying the application.

Text and Format
The **preferred word-processing package is MS-Word.** Other commonly used PC text programs and ASCII formats are accepted.
Update your data when you revise subsequent to the reviewer's or editor's decision and mark revisions clearly. Manuscripts accepted for publication are subject to **copy editing:** changes and/or questions will be marked in the manuscript, which will be returned to you with your disk and the galley proofs for checking.
Enter your text continuously flush left. Do not use any layout functions. Do not split words at the end of a line. **Do not use indentations.** Use a blank line before and a hard return at the end of paragraphs. **Arrange headings flush left.** Insert only **one space after punctuation marks.** Insert Greek letters, mathematical symbols etc. with your word-processing program. Use **boldface and italics** as well as sub- and superscript where appropriate.
Tables are part of the text and should be placed at the end of the text file. Separate the individual parts of a table by lines. Use the tabulator instead of spaces. Format operation data on one line in the same column.

Legends to illustrations are part of the text and should also be listed at the end of the text file.

Illustrations
Store illustrations as separate files: do not integrate them in your text. Export **line drawings/vector graphics** as TIF, EPS or WMF format. Use Photoshop for processing and retouching **scanned half-tone images.** Save the original scan and the processed version. Export **black and white or color images** as TIF or EPS format in their anticipated size in print. **For detailed information** on how to submit illustration data on disk please consult the leaflet or **www.karger.com/disksubmission.**

KI 02 DISK

KARGER

Fax +41 61 306 12 34
E-Mail karger@karger.ch
www.karger.com

The Journal Home Page is available at:
www.karger.com/anm

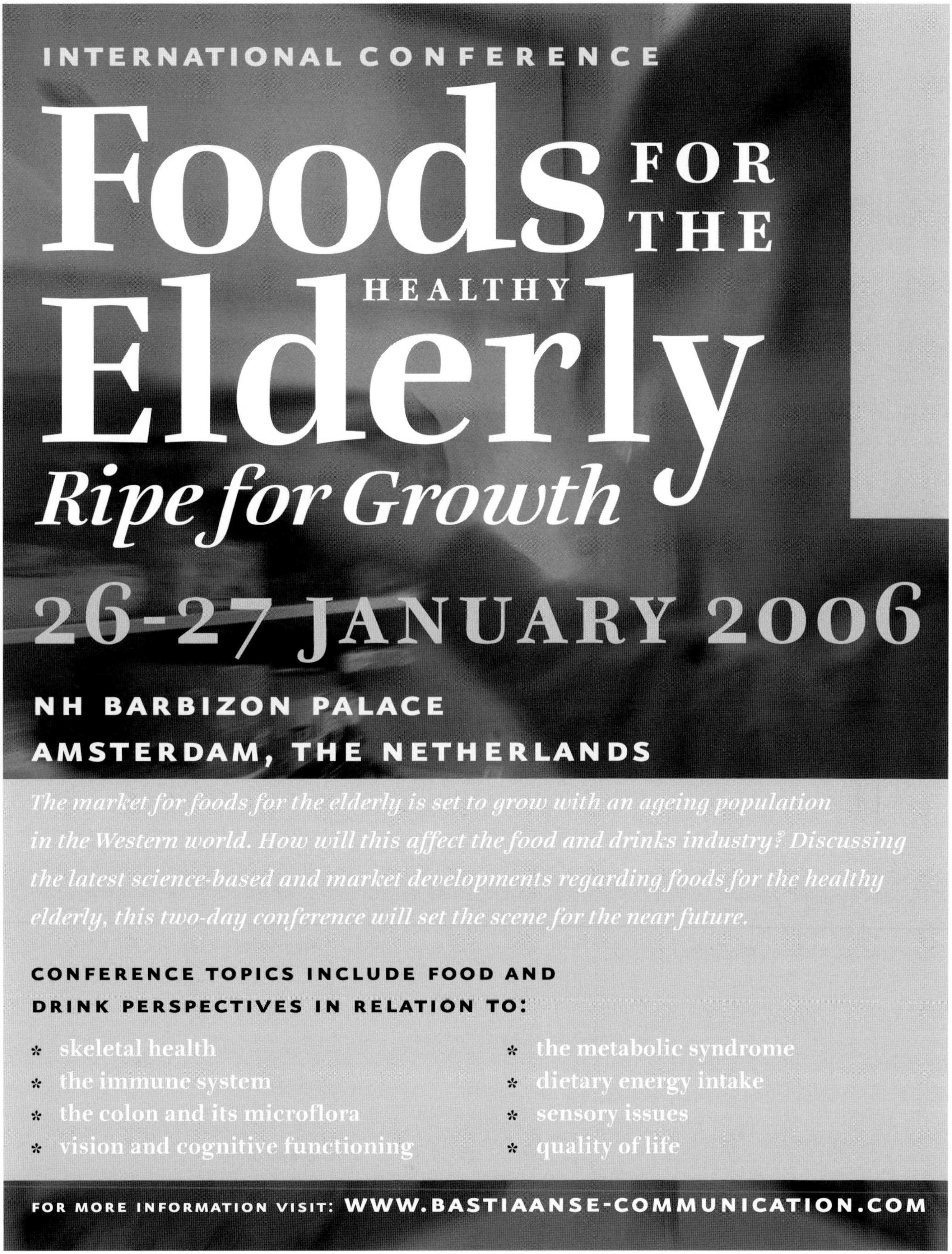
INTERNATIONAL CONFERENCE
Foods FOR THE HEALTHY Elderly
Ripe for Growth
26-27 JANUARY 2006
NH BARBIZON PALACE
AMSTERDAM, THE NETHERLANDS
The market for foods for the elderly is set to grow with an ageing population in the Western world. How will this affect the food and drinks industry? Discussing the latest science-based and market developments regarding foods for the healthy elderly, this two-day conference will set the scene for the near future.
CONFERENCE TOPICS INCLUDE FOOD AND DRINK PERSPECTIVES IN RELATION TO:
* skeletal health
* the immune system
* the colon and its microflora
* vision and cognitive functioning
* the metabolic syndrome
* dietary energy intake
* sensory issues
* quality of life
FOR MORE INFORMATION VISIT: WWW.BASTIAANSE-COMMUNICATION.COM

F 05562

The latest on the prevention, pathogenesis, diagnosis and management of this complex disease

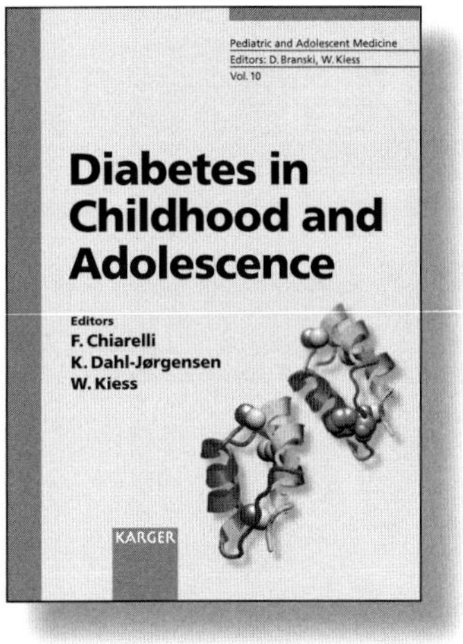

Diabetes in Childhood and Adolescence

Editors
Francesco Chiarelli
Knut Dahl-Jørgensen
Wieland Kiess

Pediatrics; Endocrinology; Metabolism; Diabetes, Genetics, Nutrition, General Medicine

Diabetes mellitus is one of the most frequent chronic diseases affecting children and adolescents. The number of young children being diagnosed with type 1 diabetes is increasing worldwide and an epidemic of type 2 diabetes already at a young age is being observed in most societies around the world.
In this book, leading experts from the USA, Europe and Israel provide a state-of-the-art summary of today's knowledge in the field of pediatric and adolescent diabetes. A number of excellent chapters deliver insight into the basic understanding of which factors contribute to or prevent the development of diabetes in young people. Other contributions provide tools for the clinician to manage the care of the child and adolescent with diabetes. In addition, knowledge from the latest scientific studies on the molecular biology of diabetes is also presented.
Providing a summary of the most recent scientific discoveries related to pediatric and adolescent diabetes, this volume will be of special interest to pediatricians, endocrinologists and health care specialists who work with children suffering from the disease.

Contents

KI 05665

www.karger.com/pam

Pediatric and Adolescent Medicine, Vol. 10
Series Editors: D. Branski, W. Kiess
ISSN 1017–5989

Diabetes in Childhood and Adolescence
Editors: Francesco Chiarelli (Chieti), Knut Dahl-Jørgensen (Oslo), Wieland Kiess (Leipzig)
VIII + 380p., 40 fig., 1 in color, 40 tab., hard cover 2005
CHF 252.– / EUR 180.– / USD 229.25
Prices subject to change
EUR price for Germany, USD price for USA only
ISBN 3–8055–7766–4

KARGER

Order Form

Please send: ______ copy/ies

Postage and handling free with prepayment

Payment:
☐ Check enclosed ☐ Please bill me

Please charge to my credit card
☐ American Express ☐ Diners ☐ Eurocard
☐ MasterCard ☐ Visa

Card No.: ____________________

Exp. date: ____________________

Orders may be placed with any bookshop, subscription agency, directly with the publisher or through a Karger distributor.

Fax: +41 61 306 12 34

S. Karger AG, P.O. Box, CH–4009 Basel (Switzerland)
E-Mail orders@karger.ch, **www.karger.com**

Name/Address: ____________________

____

____

____

____

Date: ____________________

Signature: ____________________